Myocardial Perfu
Scintigraphy

Myocardial Perfusion Scintigraphy
From Request to Report

By

Bob Bury FRCS FRCR
Consultant Radiologist

Catherine Dickinson MA PhD FRCP
Consultant Cardiologist

Karen Sheard DCR DRNI PgDip
Principal Superintendent Radiographer

Penelope Thorley PhD
Clinical Scientist

Department of Nuclear Cardiology
Leeds Teaching Hospitals Trust
Leeds
UK

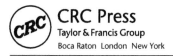

CRC Press
Taylor & Francis Group
Boca Raton London New York

CRC Press is an imprint of the
Taylor & Francis Group, an **informa** business

CRC Press
Taylor & Francis Group
6000 Broken Sound Parkway NW, Suite 300
Boca Raton, FL 33487-2742

First issued in paperback 2019

© 2004 by Taylor & Francis Group, LLC
CRC Press is an imprint of Taylor & Francis Group, an Informa business

No claim to original U.S. Government works

ISBN-13: 978-1-84184-589-0 (hbk)
ISBN-13: 978-0-367-38785-3 (pbk)

This book contains information obtained from authentic and highly regarded sources. While all reasonable efforts have been made to publish reliable data and information, neither the author[s] nor the publisher can accept any legal responsibility or liability for any errors or omissions that may be made. The publishers wish to make clear that any views or opinions expressed in this book by individual editors, authors or contributors are personal to them and do not necessarily reflect the views/opinions of the publishers. The information or guidance contained in this book is intended for use by medical, scientific or health-care professionals and is provided strictly as a supplement to the medical or other professional's own judgement, their knowledge of the patient's medical history, relevant manufacturer's instructions and the appropriate best practice guidelines. Because of the rapid advances in medical science, any information or advice on dosages, procedures or diagnoses should be independently verified. The reader is strongly urged to consult the relevant national drug formulary and the drug companies' and device or material manufacturers' printed instructions, and their websites, before administering or utilizing any of the drugs, devices or materials mentioned in this book. This book does not indicate whether a particular treatment is appropriate or suitable for a particular individual. Ultimately it is the sole responsibility of the medical professional to make his or her own professional judgements, so as to advise and treat patients appropriately. The authors and publishers have also attempted to trace the copyright holders of all material reproduced in this publication and apologize to copyright holders if permission to publish in this form has not been obtained. If any copyright material has not been acknowledged please write and let us know so we may rectify in any future reprint.

A CIP record for this book is available from the British Library.
Library of Congress Cataloging-in-Publication Data available on application

Visit the Taylor & Francis Web site at
http://www.taylorandfrancis.com

and the CRC Press Web site at
http://www.crcpress.com

Contents

Preface

Over the past 15 years, the nuclear cardiology service in Leeds has moved from a small dedicated cardiac surgery hospital to a large tertiary referral teaching centre and has grown in size from a one-camera facility into one with three cameras working full time on cardiac imaging. There have been parallel changes in staffing and working practices, to the extent that the imaging process is now almost doctor-free, with radiographers and imaging technicians stressing the patients as well as scanning them, in addition to vetting the requests and determining the protocols to be used. Medical physicists play a vital role in processing the studies, and are also present during reporting sessions, and the reporting itself is carried out by radiologists and a cardiologist. During this protracted period of change, we have learned a lot of lessons, and we thought that a book outlining our approach might be useful. For reasons outlined in the introduction and subsequent chapters, there is reason to expect that more departments will be setting up nuclear cardiology services in the UK, and although we work in a large tertiary referral centre, our reliance on the extended role of radiographers and imaging technicians is likely to be just as relevant for smaller units, if not more so.

Chapters 2 to 5 cover the logistics of service provision and will be of particular interest to radiographers and imaging technicians, although it is important for all members of the team to have an understanding of the principles involved. Chapter 6, covering the essentials of image processing, is required reading for those reporting the images as well as for the person doing the processing, and while chapter 7 does not pretend to teach the reader how to report, it does highlight important points of principle, and potential pitfalls. We also say something about the philosophy involved in producing a useful report, a topic that is not always covered in textbooks or, dare we say it, in radiology and cardiology training schemes. Chapter 8 gives the perspective of a reporting cardiologist, and therefore offers useful advice for both referrers and reporters, emphasising the need to engage with clinicians when setting up a service and ensuring that it meets clinical needs.

It is a truism that the provision of medical care is a team game, and that is certainly the case for nuclear cardiology. It is possible to run an imaging service in a vacuum, where the only contact points between referrers and service providers are the written referral and report, but this is not a professionally rewarding way to work, and results in sub-optimal patient care. Attempting to set up a nuclear cardiology facility without clinical engagement makes the job that much more difficult for those involved, and runs the risk of producing a service which fails to realise the undoubted benefits in patient outcome and cost-effectiveness which result from the appropriate use of myocardial perfusion scintigraphy. We hope that this book will help enthusiasts to build a team and set up a useful service with the minimum of pain.

BB, CD, KS, PT

Acknowledgements

The authors are grateful to the Leeds Teaching Hospitals Trust for permission to use images taken in the Nuclear Medicine Department at Leeds General Infirmary in chapters 1, 2, 4 and 5.

1

Introduction and basic principles

INTRODUCTION

Our purpose in writing this book is to provide a practical guide to setting up and running a nuclear cardiology service. A report from the National Institute for Health and Clinical Excellence (NICE) in 2003[1] illustrated the extent to which myocardial perfusion scintigraphy (MPS) is underutilised in the United Kingdom (UK). According to that report, we were performing 1200 MPS examinations per million population in 2000, with an average waiting time of 20 weeks. Expert consensus suggested that 4000 per million would be the optimal level of provision, with a maximum waiting time of 6 weeks. It was estimated that an additional 73 gamma cameras and the associated staff would be needed to meet the clinical need.

So, we would expect that there will be moves to set up nuclear cardiology services in hospitals which have not previously had access to them, and this book is intended to offer practical assistance to those involved. We have assumed that the target audience will already be providing a general nuclear medicine service, and will therefore not need any instruction in the basics of scintigraphy. There is, for example, no chapter on radiation protection or compliance with legislation, since readers will already be familiar with these topics, and we have concentrated on those areas of practice which are specific to cardiac imaging. Paradoxically, this also means that the book should be of interest to readers such as trainee cardiologists and cardiac nurses, who need to know something about nuclear cardiology but who have no background in radionuclide imaging, and no wish to wade through a lot of unwanted information on basic science and imaging technology. We also hope that the book will serve as a useful primer in nuclear cardiology for radiology trainees.

Not everyone will read the book from cover to cover, and each chapter hopefully stands alone as a guide to practice. The cardiology trainees mentioned in the previous paragraph, for example, will probably be more interested in the chapters on reporting and on the clinical role of MPS than they are in the details of service provision. As we have anticipated readers picking and choosing the sections which interest them, there is some deliberate repetition of important material and images, which we hope will not be too irritating for those who do need to read the whole book. We hope that the latter will include all radiographers, imaging technicians, medical physicists, and radiologists finding themselves involved with MPS for the first time. In all areas of radionuclide imaging, it is important for those producing the images to have an understanding of the clinical indications for imaging and the implications of the results, and for the radiologist or nuclear medicine physician doing the reporting to understand the processes which got the images on to his or her workstation. Nowhere is this more true than in nuclear cardiology, where apparent abnormalities on the images can be the direct result of problems with patient preparation, including stressing, and with image processing. Even prosaic details such as weighing and measuring the patient and, for females, recording the bra size can be critically important in assessing the relevance of imaging features.

Our aim has been to write a how-to-do-it-book, or, to be more precise, how *we* do it. In other words, this book does not review all the ways you *can* perform MPS, with a heavily referenced assessment of the evidence for and against different techniques. We describe the way we do it in Leeds in 2007, because that is what we feel competent to describe. However, over the years we have used thallium and both of the readily available technetium-labeled radiopharmaceuticals, every stress technique known to man, and any number of different imaging protocols, and the way we do it now represents a distillation of that experience, gained over 20 years or more. We do not claim that it is the only way, but it works, and appears to meet the needs of one of the largest cardiology services in Europe, so we hope that we are doing something right. We know we can still improve, and we make passing reference to some of our aspirations; for example, we want to develop a walk-in (or, rather, a wheel-in) MPS service for the acute chest pain clinic and emergency department, when resources permit.

The underlying principles behind the book, and the assumptions made, are summarised in Box. 1.1

Box 1.1   Underlying principles and assumptions

- That readers intending to set up an MPS service are already performing non-cardiac radionuclide imaging investigations in a department of nuclear medicine or radiology
- That new users will be employing technetium-labeled radiopharmaceuticals rather than thallium
- That tomographic imaging will be the norm, rather than planar
- That gated imaging will be performed wherever possible

BASIC PRINCIPLES OF MYOCARDIAL PERFUSION SCINTIGRAPHY

This section provides a brief summary of the principles underlying MPS for readers who have no background in nuclear medicine at all, and for those with general nuclear medicine experience but no previous involvement with cardiac imaging (the latter group may want to skip the first paragraph).

Nuclear medicine imaging techniques rely on the introduction of radioactive material into the body, usually by intravenous injection. The emerging gamma radiation is detected by a gamma camera (Figure 1.1), and the distribution of the material in the

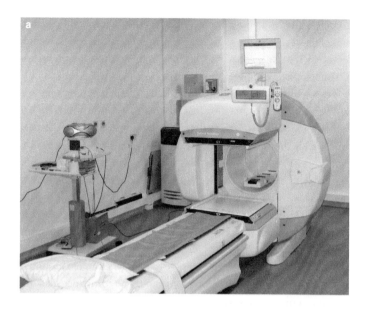

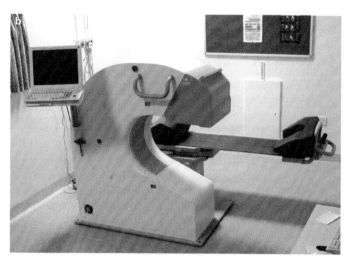

Figure 1.1 (a) Double-headed general purpose gamma camera. Each head contains a large, flat crystal of sodium iodide, which emits visible light when it absorbs a gamma ray photon. The resulting pattern of light flashes is detected and converted into a digital electronic image by a bank of photomultiplier tubes mounted on the back of the crystal. The heads rotate around the patient and acquire data from a volume which includes the heart. These data are stored in a dedicated computer and processed to produce a series of slices through the left ventricle (Figure 1.3). This particular model incorporates a low-dose computed tomography (CT) scanner in the gantry, allowing the acquisition of scintigraphic and CT images without moving the patient. These images can be superimposed, providing precise anatomical location of scintigraphic abnormalities. In nuclear cardiology practice, the CT data can be used to correct the MPS images for attenuation effects. However, this is not currently part of our routine practice. (b) Smaller footprint camera used in our nuclear cardiology department.

body is recorded digitally. The nature of the injected substance will determine which organ or physiological process is imaged. First, an appropriate chemical is chosen, which will be taken up by the tissue concerned, and this is then rendered radioactive by labeling it with a suitable isotope. The combined molecule is known as the radiopharmaceutical, and it is this which is injected into the patient. The most commonly used isotope is technetium-99m (for reasons, see Box 1.2). For MPS, we want a radiopharmaceutical which will travel in the bloodstream to the coronary arteries, and then be taken up into the cells of the myocardium. We used to use an isotope called thallium, which is treated very much like potassium by the myocardial cells, but more recently, new radiopharmaceuticals labeled with technetium have been developed. Although thallium has its strong points, these are outweighed by its disadvantages (Box 1.3), and there has been a general move to the technetium-labeled radiopharmaceuticals, which are the only ones that we will be considering in this book. Following injection, it is possible simply to position the gamma camera over the heart and acquire an image; this is known as planar imaging (Figure 1.2). However, it is also possible to rotate the camera around the patient during acquisition, and the dedicated computer can then reconstruct slices through the heart in any plane. This is tomographic imaging (Figure 1.3), and the conventions governing image display will be covered in later chapters, as will the processing of those images to obtain functional information. Tomographic imaging significantly improves the performance of MPS, and has replaced planar imaging almost completely. All the images used in this book are tomographic.

Box 1.2   Advantages of ^{99}Tc

- Readily available (from a 'generator', delivered to the department weekly, containing the longer-lived parent, molybdenum)
- Ideal half-life of 6 hours (long enough to acquire useful images; not so long that it goes on irradiating the patient and their family for days after the examination)
- Ideal energy for imaging (photons sufficiently energetic to get out of the patient; not so energetic that they pass straight through the detector)
- Chemically reactive, which means it is relatively easy to label a range of chemicals and produce radiopharmaceuticals tailored to different examinations

---

Box 1.3   Problems with thallium

- Low energy, so lots of photons are absorbed within the patient and never reach the camera, resulting in a high radiation dose, and relatively poor quality images
- Cyclotron-generated, and hence expensive and not readily available off-the-shelf in the nuclear medicine department
- Redistributes rapidly, so stress images have to be obtained immediately after the stress is applied (although redistribution can also be a relative advantage – see later chapters)

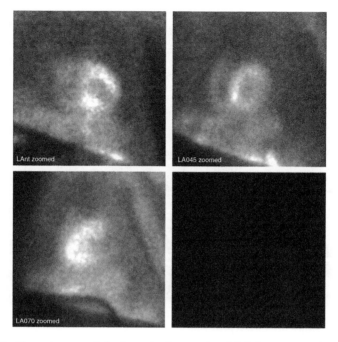

Figure 1.2 Planar images of the heart in the anterior, 45° left anterior oblique (LAO), and 70° LAO projections. These images are acquired on a single head of the gamma camera, without any movement of the gantry. Planar imaging using thallium became established as a reliable technique for the diagnosis of ischemic heart disease, but has now been almost completely replaced by the tomographic technique (Figure 1.3), since this has been shown to result in increased sensitivity and specificity. Only tomographic images are used in this book.

MPS is therefore a technique which provides a map of myocardial perfusion at the cellular level. The intention is to detect areas of myocardium at risk from ischemic damage, hopefully before it becomes irreversible. Where there is narrowing of a branch of one of the coronary arteries, perfusion of the muscle supplied by it is reduced relative to that of muscle supplied by normal vessels, and this will result in an area of relatively reduced uptake on the scan images. The technetium-labeled agents are delivered to the myocardium and taken up by intact, viable muscle cells. We image patients at stress and at rest (for reasons, see below). Once in the cells, the radiopharmaceutical stays there (unlike thallium, see Box 1.3), so as long as the injection is *administered* at peak stress, the imaging can be conducted at leisure, as the distribution of activity in the myocardium will not change with time (although the absolute amount will, due to radioactive decay). Similarly, an injection administered at rest will continue to reflect the rest distribution no matter how stressed the patient becomes before or during imaging.

At rest, the stenosed vessel may well deliver enough blood to meet the oxygen needs of the muscle, in which case the rest scan will appear normal, because approximately equal amounts of activity are delivered to all areas of the myocardium. When

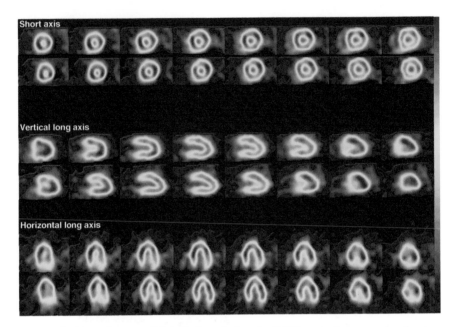

Figure 1.3 Normal myocardial perfusion scintigraphy (MPS) study demonstrating the standard image display format. The top set of images are short axis (SA) views, looking along the long axis of the left ventricle, with the anterior wall at the top, lateral wall on the right, septum on the left, and inferior wall at the bottom, apical sections on the left, to basal on the right. The stress images are displayed above the corresponding sections from the rest study. The middle rows of images are vertical long axis (VLA) views, with the anterior wall at the top, inferior at the bottom, and apex to the right, moving from the septum on the left to the lateral wall on the right. At the bottom are stress and rest horizontal long axis (HLA) views, presented with the apex at the top, lateral wall on the right, and septum on the left, moving from inferior on the left to anterior on the right.

stress increases the oxygen requirement of the myocardium, the normal response is for the vessels supplying it to dilate and deliver correspondingly more blood, and the ability of a diseased artery to respond in this way will be reduced. This is why we scan patients twice, once following injection at peak stress, and again following injection at rest. The most physiological form of stress is treadmill exercise, but the majority of our patients are unable to exercise sufficiently vigorously, and so pharmacological stress is used. This is covered in more detail in Chapter 4.

Because the stenosed vessel cannot support the increased flow demanded during stress, the increase in flow to the myocardium supplied by this vessel will be less than that to the normally perfused regions, and this will produce a perfusion defect on the stress images which is not present at rest (Figure 1.4a). It is important to understand that this defect is a *relative* one: there may actually be *more* blood going to the ischaemic area at stress than there is at rest, particularly in early disease, but the increase in flow will be less than the increase to the regions supplied by normal

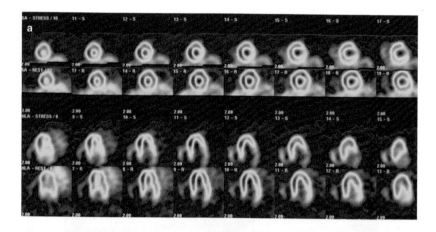

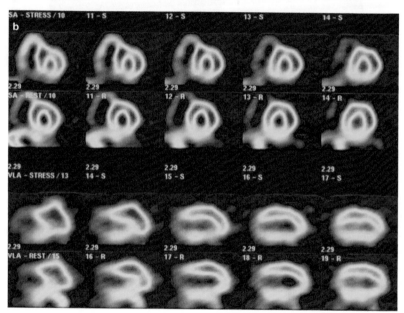

Figure 1.4 (a) Reversible defect in the lateral wall of the left ventricle. (b) Fixed defect involving the inferior wall.

vessels, and hence the *relative* defect seen on the stress images. This also explains why it is so important to optimise the level of stress achieved: modest increases in oxygen demand and hence blood flow may be capable of being met even by a stenosed vessel in early disease, and the scan will be normal. Inadequate stressing of patients will therefore reduce the sensitivity of the test.

The more severe is the limitation of flow, the greater will be the reduction of activity in the abnormal myocardium in relation to normally perfused muscle, and defects can be numerically graded to reflect this. The extent of the defect can also be

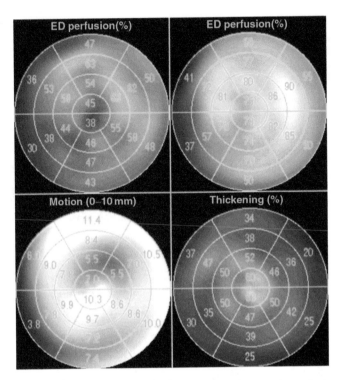

Figure 1.5 Diagram showing the 20 segment model used in semiquantitative reporting schemes.

quantified in relation to the number of segments of myocardium involved (Figure 1.5). If the reduction in blood flow becomes so critical that the myocardial cells die (myocardial infarction), there will be no uptake of radiopharmaceutical by the resulting scar tissue, and so a defect is present on stress and rest images. Thus we talk about *reversible* defects (only seen at stress – Figure 1.4a) and *fixed* defects (present at stress and rest – Figure 1.4b). Reversible defects are due to ischemia, the implication being that the muscle involved is still viable, and attempts at salvage worthwhile, whereas fixed defects are due to infarction, and so revascularization will not produce any improvement. Purists (or pedants, depending on your point of view) do not like the expression 'reversible ischaemia', arguing that the ischaemia is actually *produced* by the stress, not *reversed* by rest, and so we should actually talk about 'inducible ischaemia'. And that is true, although many of us sometimes forget to make the distinction in routine practice. Fortunately, everyone knows what we mean by reversible ischaemia.

So, the theory is:

inducible (reversible) defect = ischaemia
fixed defect = infarction

but as we shall see in subsequent chapters it is not that easy. For example, we may see fixed defects in healthy myocardium, or in chronically ischaemic muscle that is nevertheless still viable, and recognizing these and other potentially misleading appearances for what they are is the key to accurate interpretation of MPS images.

In addition to stress and rest imaging, it is good practice also to perform a gated acquisition. In gated imaging, the patient's electrocardiogram (ECG) signal is used to split each cardiac cycle into a number of equal temporal segments, and data from corresponding segments of successive cycles can be summed to produce moving images showing wall motion and thickening, and allow the calculation of quantitative parameters such as ejection fraction. As well as being useful in its own right, gating plays an important role in aiding the interpretation of the perfusion images (Chapter 7). Although the software can cope with heart rhythms which are not absolutely regular, any significant arrhythmia, particularly bigeminy and trigeminy, make gating impossible.

That was a quick guide to the principles underlying MPS. The chapters which follow will deal in more depth with the acquisition, processing and reporting of MPS studies, and also explain the clinical role of nuclear cardiology in the management of patients with ischaemic heart disease.

REFERENCE

1. National Institute for Health and Clinical Excellence. Myocardial perfusion scintigraphy for the diagnosis and management of angina and myocardial infarction. Technology Appraisal Guidance 73, November 2003.

2

Radiopharmaceuticals and equipment

CHOOSING THE BEST RADIOPHARMACEUTICAL

This section is not intended to be a comprehensive guide to radiopharmacy as there are plenty of specialist texts available. Although reference is made to thallium (^{201}Tl), it is discussed mainly to illustrate the advantages of using either of the technetium (^{99m}Tc) agents in the routine clinical assessment of patients with known or suspected coronary artery disease.

There are several issues that need to be considered when selecting the most appropriate radioactive tracer for myocardial perfusion scintigraphy (MPS). As with all nuclear medicine scans, selection of the best tracer is a compromise between the choice of physical and biological attributes, and the availability and cost (Table 2.1).

The fundamental imaging characteristics of the chosen agent should be suitable for use with modern imaging equipment, whilst delivering the lowest achievable radiation dose to the patient. When specifically considering MPS, the ideal tracer will have efficient myocardial extraction and uptake into the myocardial cells on first pass, will have stable retention during data acquisition, and, most important, will be distributed in proportion to coronary blood flow.

Currently, three MPS agents are commercially available and in widespread clinical use in the UK: thallium-201, [^{99m}Tc]sestamibi and [^{99m}Tc]tetrofosmin. These tracers can be used in a range of protocols, including:

- 1- and 2-day stress/rest or rest/stress technetium protocols
- stress/redistribution thallium protocols (either with re-injection or delayed imaging), and thallium/technetium dual isotope protocols.

THALLIUM OR TECHNETIUM?

Thallium-201 was the bastion of myocardial perfusion imaging from the late 1970s, but its popularity has been on the decline since the advent of technetium-99m imaging agents during the 1980s, and there are very few reasons to justify the continued routine clinical use of thallium in the present day.

Table 2.1 Comparison of the imaging characteristics of thallium-201, [^{99m}Tc]sestamibi and [^{99m}Tc]tetrofosmin

---

Thallium-201
- Emits predominantly mercury X-rays at 69–83 keV– relatively low energy causes problems of attenuation
- Relatively long physical half-life (73.1 hours) restricts dose that can be administered
- Cyclotron-produced so must be ordered in advance
- Uptake proportional to regional myocardial blood flow
- Redistributes in myocardium – stress images must begin immediately following stress and enables delayed redistribution images without a second injection
- Standard dose: 80 MBq (120 MBq with re-injection)
- Effective dose equivalent (ede): 14 mSv
  re-injection technique (ede): 21 mSv
- Gated SPECT and assessment of left ventricular (LV) function difficult due to poor count statistics
- Relatively low subdiaphragmatic uptake: good target-to-background ratio for early imaging

[^{99m}Tc]sestamibi and [^{99m}Tc]tetrofosmin
- Emit gamma rays at 140 keV – energy level ideal for imaging with a gamma camera
- Short physical half-life (6 hours) enables larger doses to be given
- Produced from kit and generator eluate so readily available
- Uptake proportional to regional myocardial blood flow
- Stable retention in myocardium without redistribution – allows for delayed imaging, but requires two separate injections for rest and stress studies
- Standard dose: up to 1000 MBq
- Effective dose equivalent (ede): 8–10 mSv
- Gated SPECT and assessment of LV function possible due to good count statistics
- High subdiaphragmatic uptake: imaging must be delayed for 30–60 minutes for tetrofosmin, 45–90 minutes for sestamibi

---

Apart from the obvious benefits of reduced patient dose and the ability to perform gated single photon emission computed tomography (SPECT) with assessment of left ventricular function, the technetium agents also offer a cost advantage and immediate availability. The higher energy of the technetium agents results in significantly improved count rates and resolution with subsequent superior image quality compared to thallium, and the lack of redistribution enables delayed imaging at leisure (particularly useful if the exercise laboratory is remote from the imaging equipment) and improved patient scheduling. Repeat imaging can easily be performed if there is a technical requirement to do so, for example if the images are degraded due to patient movement.

The almost 'constant' supply of technetium in the average nuclear medicine department allows for the assessment of patients admitted with acute chest pain or unstable angina. There are distinct economic advantages to using this diagnostic approach, as the number of hospital admissions can be significantly reduced, with a normal resting perfusion scan on presentation in the accident and emergency department.[1]

A substantial amount of the current literature on this subject has originated from the USA, which is hardly surprising considering the emphasis placed on delivering a healthcare system which is financially robust. But given the current climate within the National Health Service (NHS) of today, the cost-effectiveness of diagnostic and treatment pathways will most likely be subjected to more rigorous scrutiny, and may well represent the cornerstone against which cardiac imaging will be valued in the future.

Although there are compelling reasons for not using thallium in routine clinical cases, there is still significant evidence that it remains a superior tracer for the detection of viable myocardium when compared to the technetium agents.[2] However, there is a considerable difference of opinion among the nuclear cardiology fraternity about the validity of this model. The redistribution of thallium at 4 hours is unpredictable, which may lead to false 'fixed' perfusion defects, i.e. ischaemia misdiagnosed as infarction (4 hours is the standard imaging delay for a stress/redistribution imaging protocol), and where viability is the clinical question it is frequently necessary to re-image at 12 or 24 hours. Delayed imaging using thallium generally results in poor image quality, and so an alternative is to use a re-injection technique (generally 40 MBq), which is effectively a 'resting' scan, between 4 and 24 hours following the stress images. This solves the problem of incomplete redistribution seen with the 4-hour redistribution protocol with improved image quality, but with an unacceptable radiation exposure to the patient: a total administration of 120 MBq of thallium-201 results in an effective dose equivalent (ede) of 21 mSv. Given that the Administration of Radioactive Substances Advisory Committee (ARSAC)[3] recommends 'the activity for each exposure is optimised such that appropriate diagnostic information is obtained with the lowest practicable dose to the patient', it seems irresponsible to justify the routine use of thallium-201 for myocardial perfusion imaging when a technically more suitable alternative is so readily available, and where utilizing other imaging techniques is now a real alternative for most nuclear medicine departments. The issue of viability is discussed further in this chapter as well as in Chapter 5.

TECHNETIUM AGENTS – ARE THEY THE SUPERIOR ALTERNATIVE?

The decision to go with sestamibi or tetrofosmin remains one that can only be answered locally in your own department. Both agents have similar diagnostic performance and there is no discernible difference in the appearance of the reconstructed images (Figures 2.1 and 2.2).

Each agent has both advantages and disadvantages from a technical perspective which will need to be evaluated in much the same way as for any imaging agent currently in use in the nuclear medicine department.

The method of reconstitution of sestamibi is a lengthier procedure compared to tetrofosmin, as it requires boiling and cooling during preparation; however, the time taken to perform quality control procedures is shorter with sestamibi. Once reconstituted, the

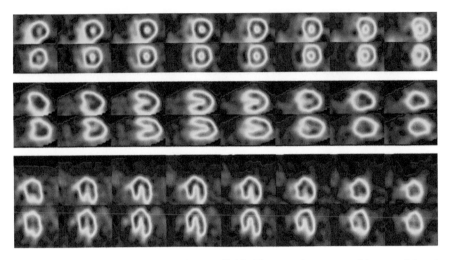

Figure 2.1   Myocardial perfusion study using ^{99m}Tc. The stress images are with sestamibi, and the rest images are with tetrofosmin.

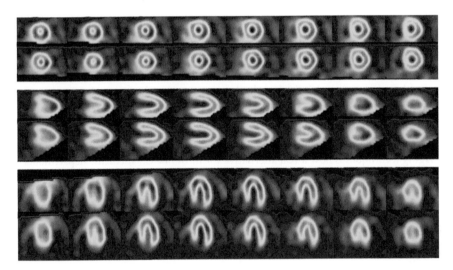

Figure 2.2   Myocardial perfusion study using ^{99m}Tc. The stress images are tetrofosmin, and the rest images are sestamibi.

'shelf life' of tetrofosmin is 2 hours longer, which may be advantageous for the single-room nuclear medicine department as it allows more flexible scheduling of patients throughout the day. Sestamibi on the other hand is also a valuable agent in parathyroid imaging, and there are economic advantages to performing these studies on the same day as the cardiac work, to maximise usage of the reconstituted vial and reduce the cost of performing isolated parathyroid studies. Although the methodology of pharmaceutical preparation may not seem to have much significance

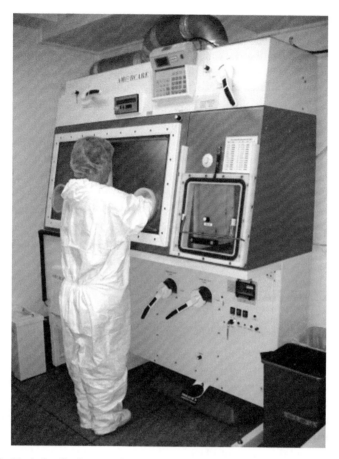

Figure 2.3 Typical radiopharmacy layout with isolator cabinet.

compared to the biological and physical characteristics of the tracers, it is highly significant if you need to introduce a change to established working practices which will require the support and cooperation of the pharmacy staff (Figure 2.3).

The major consideration is how long you are willing to wait before you start imaging following injection. Tetrofosmin is cleared from the lungs and the liver much faster than sestamibi, which results in improved resolution of early cardiac images. Imaging as early as 15 minutes has been recommended by some authors, but realistically we have found this only to be true in patients who have performed vigorous exercise on a treadmill. Further discussion about imaging protocols and optimum imaging times can be found in Chapter 5.

Our department has been biased towards the tetrofosmin agent in the past because we have the luxury of a dedicated nuclear cardiology department with three twin-headed gamma cameras available. This has enabled us to have maximum throughput of patients during a normal working day due to the shorter time from injection to imaging. Time is of the essence in our unit, and the sooner we have a patient lying underneath a gamma camera, the better. However, we currently utilise both sestamibi and tetrofosmin on a daily basis. Tetrofosmin is the agent of choice for afternoon injections, which guarantees that we can work through the day's schedule before the staff leave for home. We have also found the slight increase in delay of scanning the first 'sestamibi' patient of the day to be a bonus, as it increases the time available to spend on quality assurance, pharmacy duties, and other daily tasks. The move from a single technetium agent to combined use of sestamibi and tetrofosmin was mostly driven by economic reasons, as well as the desire to avoid putting 'all eggs in one basket' as a consequence of the limited number of suppliers of radiopharmaceuticals.

In the single-roomed general nuclear medicine department, there is the possibility of a couple of acute lung scans or a quick dynamic renal study before getting down to the nitty-gritty of cardiac imaging. Your own establishment, method of working, levels of staff, equipment, and radiopharmacy support are going to dictate which agent is best for you, as is the demand for nuclear cardiology procedures in your own hospital.

WHAT ABOUT VIABILITY?

The question of detecting viability with nuclear imaging remains one that requires answering. The technique employed depends on which feature of myocardial viability you wish to identify, namely perfusion, integrity of the cell-membrane, preservation of myocardial contractility, or metabolism. Assessment of glucose metabolism using $[^{18}F]$fluorodeoxyglucose (FDG) is well established as the gold standard. However, positron emission tomography (PET) scanners or even PET-capable gamma cameras are not to be found in every district general hospital, the technology and consumables are expensive, and the supply of FDG is still somewhat scanty in the UK. There has been considerable interest and research based around the ability to demonstrate viability using nuclear cardiology imaging techniques which have focused on the demonstration of perfusion, cell-membrane integrity, and preserved contractility:

- Many investigators (including a few in our department) have reported that the administration of nitrates before the resting injection has been shown to increase tracer uptake when using the technetium agents, and subsequently improves the detection of viable myocardium. This technique, using sublingual glyceryl trinitrate (GTN), is in routine daily use for our patients,[4] and is a common practice in many departments performing MPS.
- Routine image acquisition using a gated SPECT protocol allows an assessment of left ventricular contraction and identification of wall-motion defects. Additional gated imaging performed during an infusion of low-dose dobutamine can assess contractile reserve and differentiate viable from scarred myocardium in areas with a corresponding resting perfusion defect. This remains an area of interest and development, not just in nuclear imaging, but in magnetic resonance imaging (MRI) and echocardiography too.[5]

EQUIPMENT

The heart is quite probably the most difficult organ in the body to examine using a nuclear medicine technique! Not only does it move very frequently and quite independently of conscious thought, but also changes position within the chest cavity due to respiration, and is surrounded by tissue of varying densities. So anybody who remembers the days of planar imaging of the heart will look back and realise that SPECT was developed primarily with nuclear cardiology in mind, and that gated SPECT was the icing on the cake!

SPECT is able to accurately determine the three-dimensional distribution of the radioactive tracer within the patient, and this is especially pertinent to cardiac imaging due to the heart being a multichamber volume organ. The development of this technology has enabled myocardial perfusion imaging to grow as an essential diagnostic tool in the management of patients with coronary artery disease. Cardiac SPECT imaging overcomes the limitations of planar imaging by improving the localization and quantification of perfusion defects, as well as enhancing the ability to assess the extent and severity of perfusion abnormalities. As a result, cardiac SPECT imaging is now routinely used in nuclear medicine departments across the world.

It is obvious, therefore, that a department that wishes to set up a service to deliver cardiac imaging should have, or intend to purchase, a gamma camera that has SPECT capability. SPECT imaging is also a suitable and preferred method for investigating many other organs and specific pathologies, and therefore the purchase of this expensive piece of technology will be appealing to a wide range of nuclear medicine departments.

As for gated SPECT being the icing on the cake, there is no doubt that it is probably the most seriously underused technique in nuclear medicine today, but adds the greatest value to a diagnostic investigation that I can think of. As well as providing additional information about left ventricular function, wall motion assessment, and evaluation of cardiac size, it aids the clinician in the assessment of possible attenuation defects, and facilitates adherance to the principle of 'as low as reasonably practicable'.

Prior to the introduction of gated SPECT imaging, many patients would have needed an additional MUGA (multiple gated acquisition) scan (or radionuclide ventriculography) with its corresponding 6 mSv effective dose equivalent as part of an assessment for cardiac disease. If I was to offer one single piece of advice to a department performing or setting up a service for cardiac imaging it would be this – do gated SPECT!

TWO HEADS ARE BETTER THAN ONE?

It is perfectly feasible to perform cardiac imaging on a single-head SPECT gamma camera, but it will be necessary to impose robust methods of immobilization on the patient as data acquisition times are likely to be quite prolonged (greater than

30 minutes). Lengthy imaging times inevitably lead to an increased risk of patient movement, and images obtained where the patient has moved during the acquisition are likely to have perfusion defects, which may be interpreted as a false positive result when reconstructed, or may make interpretation very difficult (Figure 2.4).

The appearances are often characteristic of either horizontal or vertical movement, and the experienced clinician should easily recognise this artefact during image reporting (see Chapter 7). Needless to say, it would be better if the clinician never even saw the images, and the acquisition was repeated, ensuring that the patient is comfortable and other means of support are offered, or other methods of immobilization employed. Many cameras equipped for SPECT imaging now come with a range of immobilization devices, arm-rests and supports (see Chapter 5).

Dual-head gamma cameras offer shorter acquisition times, and subsequently a reduction in the number of scans repeated due to patient movement. Standard cardiac SPECT images are generally acquired with a 180° rotation, which is preferred to a 360° acquisition when using a filtered back-projection method of reconstruction. For dual-head cameras the detectors are generally configured at 90° to each other (Figure 2.5).

Choosing a circular or a non-circular orbit (elliptical or body contour) remains a contentious issue. In theory we should see improved spatial resolution of the images with a non-circular orbit due to the reduced detector to source distance. In practice, investigators have found there to be considerable variation in the resolution characteristics of the projected images, leading to an increase in image artefacts during the reconstruction process. In the end, the decision will be made for you if you do not have a gamma camera system which is capable of image acquisition using a non-circular or body contour method. Those establishments who have this 'luxury' would be wise to perform their own phantom studies before deciding on an imaging protocol.

COLLIMATOR CHOICE

The correct choice of collimator is important, as the clinical quality of the images will be affected by the selection. Due to the position of the heart within the chest cavity, and the non-circular shape of the thorax, there will be some loss of resolution in the images due to the increased distance between the source and the detector. Parallel hole collimation using a low-energy high-resolution collimator is generally recommended for cardiac SPECT imaging. Even when the target organ to detector distance is increased, good resolution is maintained with the high resolution collimator.

EQUIPMENT QUALITY ASSURANCE

As well as the standard nuclear medicine quality control tests for system uniformity, resolution, sensitivity, and energy peaking, most SPECT systems require regular centre-of-rotation (CoR) checks. Errors of alignment between the two detectors

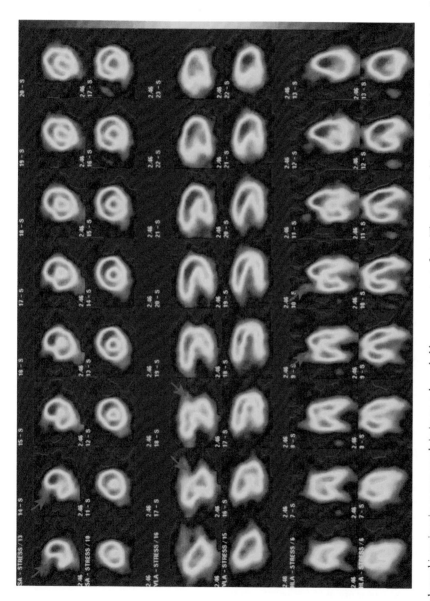

Figure 2.4 Prolonged imaging times may result in images degraded by movement artefacts. The arrows indicate a typical defect seen as a step in the contour of the ventricle (rows 1, 3 and 5). In comparison, the slices below are the repeat study in the same patient without movement artefact, and show considerable improvement in image quality (rows 2, 4 and 6).

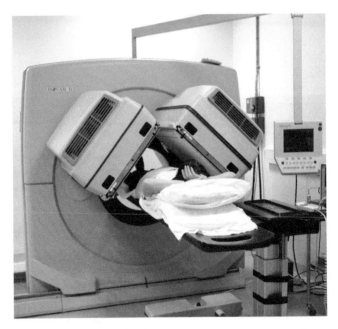

Figure 2.5 A dual-head general purpose gamma camera with the detectors in a 90° configuration for cardiac imaging. An example of a dedicated cardiac imaging system can be seen in Figure 1.1b.

cause image artefacts, and weekly or even daily checks are recommended with a variable geometry gantry. The frequency of performing quality assurance tests on the equipment will obviously be determined by the age and type of equipment and the regime that is currently in place. If you need further information or advice regarding equipment performance you should consult a specialist text or your equipment manufacturer, as this subject is outside the scope of this book.

REFERENCES

1. Knott JC, Baldey AC, Grigg LE et al. Impact of acute chest pain Tc-99m sestamibi myocardial perfusion imaging on clinical management. J Nucl Cardiol 2002; 9: 257–62.
2. Cuocolo A, Pace L, Ricciardelli B et al. Identification of viable myocardium in patients with chronic coronary artery disease: comparison of thallium-201 scintigraphy with reinjection and technetium-99m-methoxyisobutyl isonitrile. J Nucl Med 1992; 33: 505–11.
3. Administration of Radioactive Substances Advisory Committee (ARSAC). Notes for Guidance on the Clinical Administration of Radiopharmaceuticals and Use of Sealed Radioactive Sources. Section 3.2 – Activity Administered, March 2006: 12–13. (online at http://www.arsac.org.uk)
4. Thorley PJ, Sheard KL, Wright DJ, Sivananthan UM. The routine use of sublingual GTN with resting 99Tcm-tetrofosmin myocardial perfusion imaging. Nucl Med Commun 1998; 19: 937–42.
5. Bax JJ, van der Wall EE, Harbinson M. Radionuclide techniques for the assessment of myocardial viability and hibernation. Heart 2004; 90: 26–33.

3

Myocardial perfusion scintigraphy: defining its role

In 2004, cardiovascular disease (CVD) accounted for 37% of deaths in the UK. About half (49%) of all deaths from CVD are from coronary heart disease (CHD), with approximately one in five deaths in men, and one in six deaths in women. The British Heart Foundation (BHF) estimates the overall cost of CVD to the UK economy to be around £26 billion per year, which represents a huge financial burden to health and social care systems, as well as impacting upon industry and productivity in the working population.[1]

A review of the national service framework (NSF) for coronary heart disease by the Healthcare Commission in 2005 identified that there had been significant improvements in the assessment of people with suspected angina and the treatment of heart attack patients since the standards were set in March 2000.[2] The NSF outlined priorities to be achieved to improve the quality of service, tackle inconsistencies in care delivered, and reduce mortality rates from CHD over a period of 10 years. This strategy included the setting up of rapid access chest pain clinics, faster treatment of heart attack patients, and increased numbers of revascularization procedures with shorter waiting times. Implementing this strategy was likely to impact upon the major cardiac diagnostic services of coronary angiography, exercise electrocardiography (ECG), stress echocardiography and myocardial perfusion scintigraphy (MPS).

In November 2003 the National Institute for Health and Clinical Excellence (NICE) published an appraisal of the use of heart scan technology (myocardial perfusion scintigraphy) in the overall framework of the diagnosis and management of angina and myocardial infarction (Technology Appraisal Guidance 73).[3] The guidelines set a challenging target for most nuclear medicine departments, with an estimated optimum level of provision of approximately 4000 single photon emission computed tomography (SPECT) scans per million population per year, and waiting times of 6 weeks for routine scans and 1 week for urgent tests. In a national survey by the British Nuclear Cardiology Society in 2000, the estimated level of provision was 1200 SPECT scans per million and an average waiting time of 16 weeks.[4] NICE estimated the annual revenue cost of providing this increased level of activity to be around £27 million.

Our department, a dedicated nuclear cardiology facility, has struggled to meet the objectives set out in the guidelines, but we have come a long way towards achieving them. Many of the barriers encountered in service development within the National

Health Service (NHS) are finance-related – basically there is never enough money to go around, and therefore a strategy to develop or expand a nuclear cardiology service must focus on improved efficiency and new ways of working, such as skill-mix and role extension. There are usually many ways in which efficiency can be improved, but the degree to which a department can implement new ways of working is inextricably linked to existing work schedules, available resources and workforce levels.

GAINING SUPPORT

It is important to look outside your department if you are planning to implement a new myocardial perfusion imaging service in your hospital. Involvement of service-users at the planning stage is vital – there is no point in spending time and resources on the development of a new imaging technique if there is little or no demand for it. We are not suggesting that you give up at the first hint of rejection, or we would have spent the past 20 years performing bone scans, but do your homework first so that you can approach your project well informed.

Familiarise yourself with the current strategies for the investigation of patients with known or suspected coronary disease in your establishment. If you can gain the interest and support of a cardiologist or physician at this stage, you will gain insight as to whether these strategies are clinically effective. Be good to this collaborator and they will be valuable to you in the future when you want to establish stress protocols, need advice on cardiac drugs, or simply take your message about the miracle of myocardial perfusion imaging to the rest of the cardiology directorate.

At this stage it is always useful to know your MPS competitors, so investigate whether this service is available at any other hospitals within your region. If you are likely to be the sole provider you may find yourself inundated with referrals, and while this may provide you with a source of much needed income from those out-of-town referrals, it will also rapidly fill your schedule and overrun your waiting list. The key issue here is to plan your service, ensuring that you know what the level of demand is likely to be, and that you can provide the necessary level of resource to meet it.

CLINICAL INDICATIONS

A list of clinical indications for performing MPS should be available for referring clinicians and as a reference source within the department. This can also form the guidance for practitioners and/or designated and authorised specialist trained staff to justify the referral and ensure compliance with the relevant sections of the Ionising Radiation (Medical Exposure) Regulations 2000.

The referral criteria used in Leeds have expanded over the past couple of decades and now constitute a fairly exhaustive list, reflecting the high value placed on MPS

Table 3.1 Indications for myocardial perfusion scintigraphy (MPS): 1. The initial diagnosis of coronary artery disease

---

- In patients who present with typical or atypical chest pain and no proven diagnosis of CAD
- In patients with a high risk of CAD (multiple risk factors – hypertension, hypercholes- terolaemia, familial coronary disease, smoking, obesity, diabetes)
- In patients holding high-risk jobs (often referred following annual medical screening), for example: heavy goods vehicle and public service vehicle licence holders, train drivers, air- line pilots
- In situations where coronary angiography is not warranted unless MPS provides further supportive evidence of CAD (low pre-test likelihood of CAD)
- Where alternative investigations are non-diagnostic, inappropriate, or equivocal – e.g. exercise ECG testing where there is a poor workload ($<85\%$ target heart rate achieved in the absence of significant ECG changes indicative of ischaemia); where there is a coexisting mobility problem (e.g. arthritis, peripheral vascular disease, multiple sclerosis, elderly patients, etc.); where the ECG is uninterpretable (e.g. due to LBBB, RBBB, digoxin effect, etc.)
- As a preoperative evaluation in high risk patients/high risk surgical procedures (aortic aneurysms, vascular surgery, liver and renal transplantation, elderly)
- In acute chest pain

LBBB, left bundle branch block; RBBB, right bundle branch block.

Table 3.2 Indications for MPS: 2. Assessment of the severity and extent of coronary artery disease

---

- Evaluation of the functional significance of stenoses where there is angiographic evidence of coronary disease (risk stratification – the extent and severity of perfusion defects is closely related to subsequent cardiac events)
- Evaluation of acute chest pain and unstable angina
- To evaluate myocardial perfusion pre- and post-angioplasty, stent insertion, or coronary artery bypass grafting in symptomatic patients
- Where alternative investigations are non-diagnostic, inappropriate, or equivocal – e.g. exercise ECG testing where there is a poor workload ($<85\%$ target heart rate achieved in the absence of significant ECG changes indicative of ischaemia); where there is a coexisting mobility problem (e.g. arthritis, peripheral vascular disease, multiple sclero- sis, elderly patients, etc.); where the ECG is uninterpretable (e.g. due to LBBB, RBBB, digoxin effect, etc.)
- Post-infarction – mapping the extent of an infarct
- Assessment of viability
- Congenital abnormalities: children and young adults with congenital heart disease who present with typical angina pain

---

in the investigation of the patient with coronary artery disease (CAD) in our region (Tables 3.1–3.4). Not all of the criteria will be applicable to every department wish- ing to perform or currently undertaking MPS. The type of patient referred will be influenced by the existing facilities available for investigating and treating coronary

Table 3.3 Indications for MPS: 3. Assessment of chest pain in patients with angiographically normal coronary arteries

- Anginal symptoms may be caused by stress-induced microvascular disease (syndrome X), coronary spasm and muscle bridging

Table 3.4 Indications for MPS: 4. Assessment of left ventricular function

LV function analysis should be routinely performed on all patients who present for myocardial perfusion imaging (gated SPECT) where technically possible.

Advantages include:
- Evaluation of systolic function (ejection fraction, end-diastolic and end-systolic volumes) – this can be an important prognostic factor when combined with the perfusion findings
- Evaluation of wall motion abnormalities – this is particularly helpful in deciding whether fixed defects are due to attenuation
- The ability to assess function in patients where that is the primary clinical requirement, for example: renal patients being considered for transplant and patients undergoing chemotherapy with cardiotoxic drugs. Although only a gated rest scan is required in these situations, patients should undergo additional stress perfusion imaging if there is significant impairment of LV function or significant perfusion abnormality on rest imaging, usually following consultation with the referring clinician

disease in your hospital. If your patients have to travel 50 miles down the road for angiography or cardiac surgery, then the cardiologist may leave it to the treatment centre to do their own work-up on the patient, which may also be their preferred option.

Tables 3.1–3.4 categorise the four main clinical scenarios for performing MPS, and outline the criteria to which we work in Leeds. We include Table 3.4, which covers the assessment of left ventricular function, to reflect the fact that the availability of gated SPECT has now made this an integral part of any MPS study.

Historically, the exercise treadmill test was the first port of call in the investigation of patients for CAD. Many studies (notably the EMPIRE (Economics of Myocardial Perfusion Imaging in Europe) study) have shown that in the absence of documented CAD, perfusion imaging is a more reliable and cost-effective strategy.[5] The improved sensitivity and specificity of this technique (around 90% respectively) compared to treadmill testing (between 50 and 70%) gives the clinician a higher degree of confidence in the results, with fewer patients returning to the clinic with an equivocal or non-diagnostic test. This is particularly relevant in those patients where it is anticipated that the stress ECG may not give accurate or clear results, and where there is a low pre-test likelihood of CAD, as discussed in the NICE technology appraisal. Another result of the incorporation of MPS as a first-line investigation is a reduction in the number of normal diagnostic coronary angiograms being performed in the catheter laboratory. Angiography should be restricted to the investigation and treatment of patients with known disease. Not only is there an associated financial benefit from this strategy, it also offers greater patient safety, as the risk of an adverse cardiac event during MPS is very small when compared to angiography.

MPS can be a very useful tool in planning the treatment of a patient who already has a diagnosis of coronary disease. The most common reason for referral of a patient with known CAD in our unit is to assess the significance of known coronary stenoses on myocardial perfusion, enabling the cardiologist to plan the most appropriate therapy. Although coronary angiography has the status of 'gold standard' in evaluating CAD, it cannot demonstrate the effects of stenoses on perfusion at tissue level. What looks like a significant narrowing on angiography may not be producing ischaemia if there is adequate flow through collaterals. It is also the case that angiography frequently demonstrates stenoses of intermediate severity, where the cardiologist would not normally intervene unless they can be shown to be flow-limiting. Used together, angiography and MPS provide complementary anatomical and physiological information, and can ensure that any interventional treatment will target the appropriate vessels.

REFERENCES

1. British Heart Foundation Statistics Website. (online at http://www.heartstats.org)
2. Commission for Healthcare Audit and Inspection. National service framework report. Getting to the heart of it. Coronary heart disease in England: a review of progress towards national standards. Summary report, 2005.
3. National Institute for Health and Clinical Excellence. Myocardial perfusion scintigraphy for the diagnosis and management of angina and myocardial infarction. Technology Appraisal Guidance 73, November 2003.
4. Kelion AD, Anagnostopoulos C, Harbinson M, Underwood SR, Metcalfe M; British Nuclear Cardiology Society. Myocardial perfusion scintigraphy in the UK: insights from the British Nuclear Cardiology Society Survey 2000. Heart 2005; 91 (Suppl 4): iv2–5.
5. Underwood SR, Godman B, Salyani S, Ogle JR, Ell PJ. Economics of myocardial perfusion imaging in Europe - the EMPIRE study. Eur Heart J 1999; 20: 157–66.

4

Stressing the patient

There are various methods of stress suitable for myocardial perfusion scintigraphy (MPS). The 'right choice' will depend not only upon the patient's clinical condition and physical ability, but also upon the equipment, resources, skilled staff and expertise available in your department. Selecting the most suitable method for your patient is crucial, as it is essential to ensure that an optimal level of stress has been achieved if an equivocal test result is to be avoided. With this in mind, the referral card or letter should be designed to include all the relevant information that will enable the clinician or practitioner or relevant designated person to allocate the most suitable protocol to the patient (Table 4.1).

Key point

Selection of the most appropriate stress method is one of the keys to success in myocardial perfusion scintigraphy

---

On the patient's arrival in the department, a more detailed clinical history should be obtained to determine that the correct protocol has been allocated, and to ensure that there are no contraindications to performing the requested investigation. This is an important step in the pathway if your department has a lengthy waiting list, as any change in the patient's clinical condition since the referral was written may require a change in protocol. Or indeed this may be the time to discover that they are actually feeling much better since the angioplasty last week! Clearly it would be inappropriate to continue with the investigation in this type of scenario – particularly if the clinical question was to assess the coronary flow prior to a revascularization procedure. This strategy ensures that there will be compliance with the Ionising Radiation (Medical Exposure) Regulations 2000 (IRMER)[1] in justifying an exposure.

You could, of course, obtain the patient's clinical notes prior to booking an appointment – but this may be too much of a logistical nightmare if it involves more than 60 sets of case notes per week. Take time to design and tailor your own referral letter and you will gather all the relevant information and save time later on, avoiding

Table 4.1   Referrals for myocardial perfusion scintigraphy – essential required information for cardiac stress testing

Patient identification details
Name, address, date of birth, telephone no.
Hospital number/patient ID number
Referring consultant
Referring location (hospital, ward, clinic)

Clinical information
Justification for examination

Relevant medical history:
- Previous scan
- Previous myocardial infarction
- Previous cardiac surgery
- Coronary angiogram
- Interventional procedure
- Pacemaker
- Diabetic
- Hypertension
- Asthma status
- Allergies
- ECG abnormalities
- Current medication

Special considerations
Ability to exercise
Weight
Height
LMP status
Disability issues: Mobility, deafness, blindness, learning disability
Transport requirements
Communication problems (interpreter)

Clinician signature

the need to reschedule stress tests. The use of a checklist helps to minimise the chance of forgetting to ask the right questions. Our department uses a technical data sheet which follows the patient study all the way to the reporting room, recording all the relevant information at each stage.

Key point

A detailed explanation of the test beforehand increases the chance of patient compliance throughout the test and results in a more successful outcome.

This is usually an appropriate time to proffer a detailed explanation of the test to the patient. Even if your department routinely uses information leaflets, it is still important to spend time discussing the procedure, due to the large volume of information that the patient needs to assimilate. Make sure to keep the technical jargon to a minimum and use whatever means possible to ensure the patient has a good understanding of what is about to come. This patient-centred approach is paramount in ensuring compliance and cooperation throughout the investigation, and enables informed consent to be given.

Information is an important part of the patient pathway, and leaflets, posters or a patient reference folder can all be valuable tools for delivering relevant information about the procedures performed in your department and the services which you provide. The Department of Health[2] recommends providing good quality information in order to:

- improve the overall experience through increased patient confidence
- serve as a reminder of information already given
- give patients the knowledge to make informed decisions
- help patients to prepare for procedures
- improve medical outcomes and help relieve anxiety.

Make use of the 'patient information toolkit' designed by the Department of Health and available online at the National Health Service (NHS) Identity website.[2] The toolkit is a useful guide towards producing good quality information that meets the needs of the patient, and when used in conjunction with other specialist resources, can help you to ensure that your patients are adequately prepared when attending the department for MPS procedures.

WHAT IS THE BEST STRESS METHOD?

A quick literature search will trawl up many studies and papers which set out to compare treadmill testing to pharmacological stress; adenosine to dobutamine and dipyridamole; and bicycle versus treadmill for both the technetium agents and thallium imaging. There have been many conclusions drawn from a whole range of permutations of stress technique and pharmaceutical, with as many recommendations made about the best stress method for a wide spectrum of clinical scenarios. There is, however, good evidence to support a preference for treadmill or adenosine stress testing for perfusion imaging, as dobutamine and dipyridamole may underestimate the extent, severity and reversibility of defects when using [^{99m}Tc]tetrofosmin single photon emission computed tomography (SPECT) imaging.[3]

Although there are some definitive 'dos and don'ts' in stress testing and MPS (left bundle branch block jumps immediately to mind – Table 4.2), there is no doubt that the most appropriate, and certainly the best stress method is the one that your department

Table 4.2   Clinical situations requiring specific stress protocols

---

Dynamic exercise (treadmill or bicycle ergometer)
Treadmill or bicycle ergometer
Anomalous coronary arteries
Muscle bridging
Microvascular disease

Vasodilator – adenosine or dipyridamole
LBBB or paced rhythm
Aortic stenosis
Wolff–Parkinson–White syndrome

LBBB, left bundle branch block.

has the skills, knowledge, support, facilities and funding to perform, and the one which meets the demands of the service that you are required to provide (Table 4.2).

SKILLS MIX

We are extremely fortunate in our department to have the facilities and technical expertise available to offer any method of stress testing to the patient. In a routine week we are able to perform a mixture of adenosine, dobutamine, treadmill and combined adenosine/treadmill stress testing, although today we lean heavily towards performing adenosine stress (around 90% of the workload). Only 10 years ago the picture looked very different, with an almost 50/50 split between treadmill testing and pharmacological challenge with dobutamine. The change was entirely driven by two issues, which are likely to be a major influence in any department performing or about to undertake MPS:

- long waiting lists
- access to medical cover for stress testing.

Widespread clinical acceptance and confidence in the diagnostic reliability of MPS within our region around 10 years ago presented us with escalating numbers of referrals. Our stress protocol strategy was totally inadequate as it was completely at the mercy of a rigid scheduling system, and dependent upon the support and input of other clinical groups such as exercise electrocardiogram (ECG) technicians and medical staff. The only way forward was to take control of the entire service within our own department through role extension and skills mix (Table 4.3). This approach to service development is relatively commonplace in the NHS today, but was fairly radical for our team at the time, as there was little guidance and no defined training pathways or competency assessment models available.

The process of introducing skills mix was underpinned by rigorous protocols, making use of the training opportunities available locally and, most important, establishing

Table 4.3 Useful skills for stress testing

Skills mix

- ECG recording and interpretation
- Treadmill testing
- Administration of pharmacological stress agents
- Taking a clinical history

a robust system of regular review and audit of clinical practice. This methodology is central to the Royal College of Radiologists' publication 'Skills Mix in Clinical Radiology',[4] and this guidance is the platform upon which we have continued to build. Today the service is managed by a skilled team of ILS (immediate life support) trained advanced practitioner radiographers who plan, perform and supervise around 75 stress tests for MPS per week. They are supported by consultants in radiology and cardiology as well as specialist registrars seconded to the department for training purposes.

If you are just about to embark upon a new cardiac service, you are probably not going to be in a position to offer a technician- or radiographer-led service from the outset. Many departments still rely heavily upon cardiac technicians, specialist nurses and medical staff, as they do not have the personnel who are adequately skilled at ECG interpretation. Involve your local ECG or cardiology department in your service development to tap into their expertise, and this may provide you with a pathway towards training opportunities. An excellent underpinning knowledge of ECG analysis is essential if you wish to produce a high-quality stress service which is safe for patients.

Whatever method of stress you choose it is essential that it is performed by appropriately trained healthcare staff in possession of a current certificate in immediate life support (ILS) and working within local departmental, hospital, and/or national guidelines and policy. If it is possible to access and train staff in advanced life support (ALS), then this is a preferable option. Otherwise, personnel who are ALS trained or a physician with appropriate experience in cardiovascular stress should be readily available for assistance if required in an emergency. A statement or strategy outlining suitable training, core knowledge and experience should be developed locally as a method of determining training requirements, and assessing competency and skills.

SELECTING A STRESS METHOD

Dynamic exercise using a treadmill or bicycle has historically been the method of choice in the routine assessment of patients for coronary artery disease (CAD) due to its widespread availability in many hospitals throughout the UK and its relatively low cost. However, there are significant limitations to this technique, with an overall sensitivity and specificity for CAD of about 63% and 74% respectively.[5] The addition of myocardial perfusion imaging can result in a significant increase in the diagnostic accuracy of this method of cardiac assessment, with sensitivity and specificity reported as high as 96% and 91% respectively for exercise studies using tetrofosmin.[6]

Advocates of dynamic stress testing will argue that it is a superior method when combined with myocardial perfusion scintigraphy, compared to pharmacological stimulation, because it is physiological, and also enables simultaneous observation of the patient's exercise tolerance and markers of ischaemia (symptoms, ECG changes, blood pressure response). In addition, physiological exercise leads to improved image quality due to increased myocardial counts compared to pharmacological stress,[3] and reduced uptake of the tracer in the splanchnic organs for both thallium and technetium agents.

In an ideal world, all patients attending for MPS in your department would undergo a treadmill stress test. But things are frequently far from ideal – many patients are barely capable of walking to the treatment room, making 9 minutes of a Bruce protocol on the treadmill an unachievable option, or the treadmill may be located on the other side of the hospital, or is only available on a Tuesday afternoon during your peak bone imaging session. Having a treadmill stress room within the nuclear medicine department is obviously the most favourable situation, even more so if the nuclear medicine staff have the skills to operate it. Multidisciplinary team working and smart negotiation will be the order of the day if you have neither. As many technician-based services are currently suffering from recruitment and retention problems in the NHS, the option to train your own staff remains an attractive one. If pharmacological challenge is the preferred or only feasible option, then appropriate protocols should be drawn up for adenosine (or dipyridamole) and dobutamine stress, as there will most likely be patient exclusions for each of these agents. As previously stated, the preferred choice will invariably be linked to the resources that are available and dictated by the patient's clinical presentation and medical history, but it is important to give consideration to the evidence that supports either treadmill testing or pharmacological stress with adenosine as superior stress methods.

CONTRAINDICATIONS

Chapter 3 discussed the many benefits of and indications for MPS, but on the downside there are almost as many reasons not to perform MPS. There are a number of specific situations and conditions in which cardiac stress testing has a high likelihood of causing harm to a person, so any department undertaking MPS should ensure that they have well documented protocols in place to ensure that patients who may be at risk are excluded. If your hospital has a stress ECG laboratory, they will most certainly be working within guidelines and protocols which specify the absolute and relative contraindications to dynamic stress testing (Table 4.4). So do not waste time reinventing the wheel; ask them for a copy and adapt it for the MPS service.

The absolute contraindications are fairly standard, and expressly prohibit performing a stress test due to the high risk to the patient. A relative contraindication does not rule out performing a procedure as long as there has been a risk/benefit assessment, or consultation with the referring clinician. Other contraindications to

Table 4.4   Absolute and relative contraindications to stress testing in myocardial perfusion scintigraphy

___

Dynamic stress – treadmill or bicycle ergometer

Absolute contraindications
- Recent acute myocardial infarction (MI)
- Aortic stenosis or hypertrophic obstructive cardiomyopathy
- Unstable angina
- Left main stem disease
- Uncontrolled symptomatic heart failure
- Severe hypertension: systolic blood pressure (BP) > 180 mmHg; diastolic BP > 100 mmHg
- Recent history of ventricular arrhythmias, e.g. VF or VT
- Recent pulmonary embolism
- Acute endocarditis, myocarditis or pericarditis
- Thrombophlebitis or active deep vein thrombosis (DVT)

Relative contraindications
- Left bundle branch block (LBBB)
- Right bundle branch block (RBBB)
- Ventricular paced rhythms
- Atrial fibrillation
- Physical or mental disability
- Digoxin use

Vasodilator stress – adenosine and dipyridamole

Absolute contraindications
- Asthma – history of significant bronchospasm
- Wheeze on chest auscultation at time of stress test
- Heart block > first degree
- Sick sinus syndrome without pacemaker
- Hypotension: systolic blood pressure < 90 mmHg
- Known hypersensitivity to adenosine or dipyridamole
- Xanthine intake in the last 12 hours or dipyridamole use in the last 24 hours

Relative contraindications
- Recent acute MI
- Bradycardia < 40 beats/minute

Inotropic stress – dobutamine ± atropine

Absolute contraindications
- As for dynamic stress above
- Known hypersensitivity to dobutamine
- Hypokalaemia

Relative contraindications
- LBBB and RBBB as above
- Ventricular paced rhythms
- Atrial fibrillation

___

VF, ventricular fibrillation; VT, ventricular tachycardia.

treadmill stress testing specifically are related to the patient's physical capability and willingness to perform dynamic exercise rather than its potential to do harm.

Left bundle branch block (LBBB) and paced rhythms are known to produce reversible septal defects and abnormal septal wall motion on MPS scans, producing a false positive result when using physical stress.[7] The phenomenon has been reported as being rate-related, ruling out dobutamine as an alternative stress method also. Current guidelines recommend MPS with adenosine as the method of stress in this group of patients. Careful consideration has to be given to the presence of a reversible septal defect at the reporting stage if it has been necessary to use a stress method other than a coronary vasodilator in the presence of LBBB. Right bundle branch block (RBBB) has also been reported to induce perfusion defects in the inferior territory, although the evidence is not as well validated as with LBBB.

If there is any doubt that the patient will be capable of attaining a minimum level of exercise of at least 85% of their maximum predicted heart rate due to medical or physical incapability, age, or poor fitness level, or if the patient is unable to understand what is required of them (e.g. due to a learning disability), then pharmacological stress is the best option.

If your department has a choice of stress method available, it is useful to design a flow chart which makes allocation of the most appropriate protocol a more robust process. Making it available to referring clinicians will help them to understand the protocol pathways in the department, as well as helping to ensure the referral contains appropriate and relevant clinical information. Tables 4.5–4.7 outline the indications for each stress method with treadmill stress as the starting point. If any of the contraindications apply, the next stress method should be selected, and the patient's suitability for that stress method assessed.

If the patient has any of the contraindications, or is unable to meet the indications required for treadmill testing, then the next choice should be adenosine stress, with or without physical challenge as appropriate (Table 4.6). The same indications and contraindications for adenosine can be applied to pharmacological stress with dipyridamole, if this is the vasodilator drug of choice.

In the event that the patient is unable to meet the criteria for either the treadmill or adenosine protocol, then dobutamine remains the only option (Table 4.7). This can be rather 'tricky' on occasion, as many of the contraindications to treadmill testing also apply to dobutamine stress.

The most common reason for not performing adenosine stress is a history of asthma. This can be quite problematic, as many patients have been 'told' they have asthma, or indeed present to the department on bronchodilator therapy having never had an appropriate evaluation of lung function. Enlisting your local respiratory function laboratory, specialist respiratory nurse, or chest physician for advice and support is useful if you wish to avoid performing a significant number of dobutamine stress tests. If there are contraindications to the use of dobutamine then it is all the more important to determine whether the patient truly has a diagnosis of asthma, if you

Table 4.5   Indications and contraindications for treadmill stress testing

Indications	Contraindications
• All patients referred for MPS will undergo stress testing by treadmill (Bruce protocol) unless any of the contraindications apply • The patient must be able to exercise to an acceptable workload (at least 85% of maximum predicted heart rate) • Dynamic exercise is the recommended stress method for patients with suspected or known anomalous coronary arteries, muscle bridging or microvascular disease (*BNMS Guidelines*)	Acute MI, unstable angina LV outflow obstruction (AS/HOCM) Left main stem disease Severe hypertension Physical/mental impairment LBBB/RBBB Arrhythmias/atrial fibrillation Acute myocarditis/pericarditis Pacemaker in situ Heart failure Pulmonary embolism DVT

BNMS, British Nuclear Medicine Society; LV, left ventricular; AS, aortic stenosis; HOCM, hypertrophic obstructive cardiomyopathy.

Table 4.6   Indications and contraindications for adenosine stress testing

Indications	Contraindications
• All patients unable to perform or unsuitable for a treadmill stress test should undergo a pharmacological stress test using adenosine unless any of the contraindications apply • If the patient is capable of exercise on a treadmill at a submaximal level, then a combined adenosine/treadmill (or bicycle ergometer) protocol can be used with the most appropriate exercise protocol for the patient, e.g. limited Bruce, modified Bruce, or Naughton (unless any of the contraindications to treadmill testing apply) • Adenosine without treadmill is the stress method of choice for patients with a pacemaker or LBBB on ECG	Recent MI, unstable angina Asthma Heart block > first degree Sick sinus syndrome without pacemaker Hypotension: systolic blood pressure < 90 mmHg Known hypersensitivity to adenosine Dipyridamole use (within 24 hours) Xanthine use (within 12 hours)

Table 4.7   Indications and contraindications for dobutamine stress testing

Indications	Contraindications
• All patients unable to perform a treadmill exercise stress test and where adenosine is contraindicated will undergo a dobutamine stress test	Acute MI, unstable angina
	LV outflow obstruction (AS/HOCM)
	Left main stem disease
	Severe hypertension
	LBBB
	Arrhythmias/atrial fibrillation
	Acute myocarditis/pericarditis
	Pacemaker in situ
	Heart failure
	Hypokalaemia

wish to avoid returning them to the referring clinician without a result. This will occasionally be the case in a small number of patients who may require referral to alternative imaging departments for further evaluation.

Recent evidence suggests that a history of asthma or chronic obstructive airway disease need not necessarily exclude a patient from an adenosine stress test if the patient has well-controlled disease or mild to moderate symptoms. The prophylactic use of an inhaled bronchodilator (e.g. salbutamol) prior to the administration of a titrated adenosine infusion has been shown to result in a safe procedure in patients with a history of mild well-controlled asthma or chronic obstructive pulmonary disease (COPD).[8] This is a procedure that our department now currently employs without a discernible increase in the number of patients experiencing manifest bronchospasm requiring nebulizer therapy, compared to earlier protocols, where all patients with a history of asthma and chronic COPD were excluded.

Again we cannot overemphasise the importance of following departmental procedures and guidelines for ensuring that your patient has been allocated the most appropriate stress protocol – not 'believing' your patient to be asthmatic is not an adequate reason. Ensure that you have sound evidence which supports your decision. And as with all decisions of this caliber, refer to the clinical head of department, or the clinician with responsibility, where there is any doubt or possibility of risk to the patient. In considering the merits of vasodilator stress, it would be pertinent to mention dipyridamole at this juncture. It has been almost 20 years since we routinely used this method of stress, and we would strongly resist any moves to reinstate it as a potential stress method in our department. Despite the fact that it is by far the cheapest available pharmacological stress agent available, it is also by far the worst vasodilator stress agent for inducing prolonged side-effects, due to its relatively long half-life. In the busy nuclear medicine department there is little or no time available for attending patients for lengthy periods when they continue to experience severe adverse effects following an infusion of dipyridamole. The general department undertaking only half a dozen stress tests per week may be influenced by the financial attractions of this drug, but be warned that you will need to have good nursing and medical back-up to provide post-stress care for your patients, and a ready supply of aminophylline to deal with those resistant prolonged side-effects. Data suggest comparable sensitivity with adenosine, although specificity may be lower, as maximal vasodilatation may not be achieved in all patients with dipyridamole.[9]

As previously noted, our MPS service uses predominantly adenosine stress at the present time. The basis for this lies in the constant requirement to adapt and respond to the challenge of a changing NHS environment. Greater patient choice, government targets and initiatives, and the promise to almost 'wipe out' waiting lists means we must constantly reassess and redesign our services to keep apace of the changes. This for us has meant increasing the number of studies performed in a day, which could only be achieved if the majority of the stress tests were performed using adenosine, which brings us nicely back to the beginning of this chapter.

Key point

There is no doubt that the most appropriate, and certainly the best stress method is the one that your department has the skills, knowledge, support, facilities and funding to perform, and the one which meets the demands of the service that your are required to provide

---

FACILITIES

As well as providing skilled and experienced staff, it is equally important to ensure that appropriate facilities are available for whatever method of stress you are going to provide (Figure 4.1). The location of the treatment or stress room is vital, as it is crucial that assistance can reach you quickly when summoned in an emergency. An alarm-call system, or at the very least a telephone within the room, is an essential requirement. Routine testing of the alarm system should take place on a regular basis as well as random activation of the alarm, to ensure that there is a prompt reaction from staff when required. Recognition of the alarm should be included in the induction plan for new staff in the department.

Rooms should be light and air-conditioned with good temperature control, and sufficiently large to allow resuscitation procedures to be performed without hindrance. Provision should be made for immediate access to resuscitation equipment

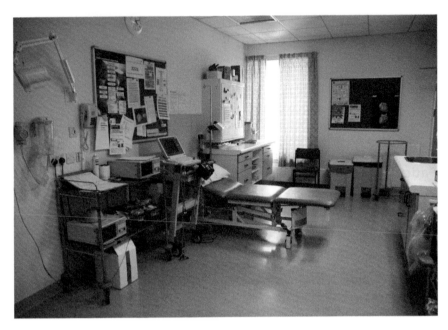

Figure 4.1 A treatment room suitable for pharmacological cardiac stress testing. The resuscitation equipment, an integral part of the stress-testing service, is just visible in the bottom right of the image and is in close proximity to the patient.

and drugs to ensure that there is a rapid response in the event of cardiopulmonary arrest, and there should be a schedule to ensure that regular checks and cleaning of all equipment and drugs take place.

Your establishment should have a resuscitation committee who are responsible for ensuring standardization of the layout of equipment and drugs throughout the institution. They are responsible for providing training and advice, and will support you in undertaking a risk assessment in your department prior to commencing your cardiac stress testing service.

USEFUL GUIDELINES

There is a multitude of procedure guidelines which can be accessed, and they form a useful resource to aid in protocol and policy development as you prepare for the development of a stress myocardial perfusion imaging service:

- British Nuclear Cardiology Society – http://www.bncs.org.uk
- British Cardiovascular Society – http://www.bcs.com
- Resuscitation Council (UK) – http://www.resus.org.uk

- European Society of Cardiology – http://www.escardio.org
- European Association of Nuclear Medicine – http://www.eanm.org
- Society of Nuclear Medicine – http://www.snm.org
- American Society of Nuclear Cardiology – http://www.asnc.org to mention but a few.

TREADMILL STRESS PROCEDURE

Patient preparation

1. *Stop beta blockers and calcium channel antagonists for 48 hours; and aminophylline, theophylline, other methylxanthines, and dipyridamole for 24 hours before the test.* Drugs that prevent a normal physiological heart rate response to exercise (i.e. beta blockers and calcium channel antagonists) should be withdrawn for at least 48 hours prior to the test unless medically contraindicated, e.g. refractory hypertension. Routinely preparing the patient for adenosine stress by stopping dipyridamole, aminophylline, theophylline and other methylxanthines for 24 hours prior to the stress scan (see adenosine protocol below) removes the need to cancel and rebook a new stress test appointment if the patient is unsuitable for a treadmill test, or fails to achieve the necessary workload.

Key point

Enlist the help of your pharmacy department to compile a list of the brand names of the most commonly dispensed beta blockers and calcium channel antagonists at your establishment to include with your patient information leaflet

---

2. *Stop caffeine-containing food, drinks and drugs for 12 hours before the test.* As above, this step is required prior to the administration of adenosine if required in the event of a failed treadmill test (see adenosine protocol).
3. *Dress in clothes and footwear suitable for exercise.* Make use of the patient information leaflet again to suggest appropriate clothing and footwear. This is particularly important for female patients where 'separates' are preferable to a dress, and trainers or flat shoes are infinitely preferable to high-heeled shoes. A supply of front-fastening gowns helps your female patients to retain their dignity during treadmill stress testing.
4. *Starve for 4 hours.* Although there is no good evidence to suggest that starving results in improved uptake of tracer, increased image quality, or decreased subdiaphragmatic activity, it is a policy we have adopted in our department. This is

primarily because nausea and vomiting following a stress test are more common in patients who have recently eaten. Reducing the incidence of nausea and vomiting helps to prevent significant reflux of activity into the stomach from the duodenum. This is particularly important for the technetium tracers, which are excreted via the hepatobiliary route, as the presence of activity in the stomach may result in severe degradation of the images. Patients who are known to have a hiatus hernia or gastro-oesophageal reflux should be given metoclopramide to promote gastric emptying and prevent reflux of radiopharmaceutical into the stomach, as activity within the thoracic region can significantly impair image quality. Metoclopramide should be given as a single oral 10-mg dose immediately following the injection of the radioactive tracer, paying particular attention to the specific drug interaction warnings. There is little evidence to suggest that the administration of metoclopramide results in the reduction of generalised abdominal activity, and therefore the routine use of metoclopramide to aid clearance of bowel activity is not recommended.[10]

5. *Weigh the patient,* to calculate the radiopharmaceutical dose required. A note of this value should be made on the technical data sheet, as it is a useful reference at the reporting stage when considering attenuation and image quality issues. Other patient statistics that are of value, namely height and additionally bra size in females, should also be recorded.

6. *Carry out a medical history check.* A check to ensure that the patient has been allocated to the correct protocol and that there are no recent medical problems or contraindications to proceeding with the stress test confirms that the administration of a radiopharmaceutical is properly justified.

7. *Give a detailed explanation of the procedure and obtain consent.* On arrival in the department, a detailed explanation of the procedure should always be given to the patient, outlining possible side-effects and complications. Use this opportunity to confirm that they have complied with the preparation required for the procedure, again entering relevant responses onto the technical data sheet. It is important to write down relevant information at the time it is given to you, as it is easy to forget to do it later, and the information may then not be disclosed to the rest of the team. A check of the pregnancy status of female patients of child-bearing age should be made, and a signature obtained on a disclosure form in line with local procedures. Verbal or written consent should be obtained as dictated by local policy.

Mechanism and protocol (Table 4.8)

The Bruce protocol is an extensively validated technique and is the one in most common use for stress testing. The protocol comprises seven stages with each stage lasting 3 minutes. Stage 1 is at a speed of 1.7 mph (2.7 km/h) with a 10% incline, and the energy expenditure is estimated to be 4.8 metabolic equivalents (METs). The metabolic equivalent value gives an indication of the workload that the patient has achieved, but we have not found it to be a particularly useful indicator during MPS studies.

Table 4.8   Treadmill protocol

- Record a baseline 12-lead ECG and repeat at the end of each stage throughout the test. Maintain observation of the real-time ECG display to monitor ST segment and T-wave changes and detect arrhythmias

- Record a baseline blood pressure (BP) and heart rate (HR) and at the end of each exercise stage. Abnormal findings of any of the baseline values (ECG, BP and HR) will necessitate a reevaluation of the stress protocol

- Insert intravenous (IV) cannula – back of hand opposite the BP cuff – and flush with sodium chloride 0.9% injection to ensure patency. Attach an extension with a three-way connector to aid the injection and minimise the risk of a spill and contamination during administration at peak exercise

- Exercise using a standard Bruce protocol to a minimum of 85% maximum predicted heart rate (MPHR) or until the patient has ECG evidence of ischaemia (ST segment depression) or becomes symptom limited

- Inject radiopharmaceutical at peak stress and continue to exercise for 1–2 minutes post-injection (refer to Chapter 5 for dose schedule)

- Allow the patient to continue walking, if capable, for up to 2 minutes in the recovery phase to 'cool down'

- Continue to monitor ECG, BP and HR parameters during recovery until they return close to baseline, or until any ischaemic changes recover

- Record the exercise duration, symptoms, ECG changes and reason for stopping the test

---

Key point

Workload is measured in metabolic equivalents (METs) and is a reflection of oxygen consumption and hence energy use
   1 MET is 3.5 ml oxygen/kg per minute, which is the oxygen consumption of an average individual at rest

---

The entire protocol lasts for 21 minutes, but this is a target that few patients attain, and generally speaking a good level of stress can be achieved after 9–12 minutes. As many patients are unaccustomed to performing exercise at this level, the most common reason for terminating the test remains fatigue and breathlessness. Plenty of support and encouragement will help the patient to achieve more than they believe they are capable of – just ensure that you keep one eye on the ECG monitor at all times.

Determining the appropriate point at which to inject the radiopharmaceutical can be quite challenging, but does become easier with experience. As a rule of thumb, do not inject if the heart rate is less than 85% of the maximum predicted heart rate

(MPHR) unless there is significant evidence of myocardial ischaemia present on the ECG (ST segment depression of >2 mm) combined with exercise-limiting symptoms. A suboptimal exercise test at this stage is likely to result in a suboptimal result at the reporting stage.

Key point
Maximum predicted heart rate (MPHR): calculated as 220 minus the patient's age (210 in women) Achieving a minimum of 85% of MPHR indicates a satisfactory heart rate response

Be wary of false positive ECG changes such as ST depression in patients taking digoxin, or in those with Wolff–Parkinson–White syndrome with manifest preexcitation. Adenosine is the preferred stress method in both of these clinical situations.

If the patient has managed to exercise to at least 85% MPHR, then there is a good probability that ischaemic changes will be detected if present during perfusion imaging. The evidence for this comes from the 'ischaemic cascade' as presented by Nesto and Kowalchuk[11] which describes the sequence of pathophysiological events following the onset of an ischaemic event. The cascade shows that abnormalities of perfusion occur much earlier than ECG changes, left ventricular dysfunction, or anginal chest pain, and explains why perfusion imaging has greater sensitivity for the detection of coronary artery disease than other diagnostic techniques, even at submaximal levels of stress. Even allowing for this, achieving 85% MPHR should not be seen as an indication for termination of the stress test alone, but should always be accompanied by other symptom limiting indicators such as chest pain, ECG evidence of ischaemia, dyspnoea and fatigue. Patients who fail to achieve 85% MPHR due to poor fitness levels should undergo pharmacological stress testing instead.

It may be necessary to terminate the test prematurely (Table 4.9) if the patient develops any signs or symptoms indicative of severe ischaemia, electrical disturbance or heart failure, and it is important that a senior and experienced member of staff makes a decision whether to inject the activity at this point, as the patient's clinical needs will take priority.

It is recommended to continue walking for 1–2 minutes after the radiopharmaceutical has been administered to allow optimal tracer clearance from the blood. In addition, reducing the level of exercise to a lower stage immediately following the injection may help the patient if they are finding it difficult to continue walking. Once the treadmill enters the recovery phase, the patient should be allowed to continue walking on the flat at a reduced speed for a couple of minutes as a 'cool-down' period. This helps the heart rate and breathing return towards normal gradually, and can help avoid fainting or dizziness, which can result from blood pooling in the large

Table 4.9 Reasons for terminating treadmill test

ECG criteria
- ST segment depression >3 mm
- ST segment elevation in non-Q wave leads
- Serious arrhythmias: VF, VT, AF, sustained SVT, frequent ventricular extrasystoles, multifocal ventricular extrasystoles
- Second- or third-degree heart block
- Symptomatic bradycardia

Signs and symptoms
- Fall in BP: to 20 mm below baseline or more than 20% from previous stage recording
- Rise in BP: systolic >240 mmHg; diastolic >120 mmHg
- Chest pain
- Severe fatigue
- Dyspnoea
- Central nervous system symptoms: ataxia, dizziness or near syncope

AF, atrial fibrillation; SVT, supraventricular tachycardia.

muscles of the legs when vigorous activity is stopped suddenly. Cardiac monitoring should be continued until the heart rate and blood pressure return close to baseline values, or until any stress induced ECG abnormalities or symptoms have resolved. A close watch should be kept on the ECG and the patient in the post-stress phase, as many arrhythmias and other symptoms can occur during recovery. The cannula should remain in situ until the end of the test in case it is necessary to administer emergency drugs, and indeed can remain in place until after the imaging if you have any concerns about the patient's clinical status.

A bicycle ergometer may also be used for stress testing, and a typical protocol generally begins with a low workload of 25 watts, followed by increases of 25 watts every 2 or 3 minutes until an end-point is achieved. Many patients find using a bicycle quite difficult due to leg fatigue, and in our experience a greater proportion of stress tests are submaximal compared to treadmill stress. If this is your only option, then a combined exercise–adenosine protocol may be a better option.

ADENOSINE (AND DIPYRIDAMOLE) STRESS PROCEDURE

Patient preparation

1. *Stop aminophylline, theophylline, other methylxanthines, and dipyridamole for 24 hours before the test.* Aminophylline, theophylline, caffeine and other methylxanthines are competitive adenosine antagonists and should be avoided for 24 hours prior to the test, as the vasoactive effects of adenosine will be inhibited. Adenosine can be safely administered in the presence of other cardioactive drugs (beta blockers, digitalis, and calcium channel antagonists); however, due to the potential additive effect on the sinoatrial (SA) and atrioventricular (AV) nodes, adenosine

should be used with caution in patients who have bradycardia due to concomitant drug therapy (e.g. beta blockers).

Dipyridamole augments the action of adenosine and should always be discontinued for 24 hours prior to the investigation.

2. *Stop caffeine-containing food, drinks and drugs for 12 hours before the test.* Food and drinks containing caffeine (tea, coffee, chocolate, cola and some other soft drinks) should be avoided for at least 12 hours prior to the test. Some drugs, particularly cold and flu remedies, and some pain killers available over the counter, may also contain caffeine. Information sheets or appointment letters should also instruct patients to avoid decaffeinated products, which frequently contain some caffeine, as opposed to caffeine-free products, which do not.

3. *Starve for 4 hours.* As above for the treadmill test, all patients are routinely starved for 4 hours.

4. *Weigh the patient and calculate adenosine dose and infusion rate.* Weigh the patient to calculate the radiopharmaceutical dose required and to determine the adenosine dose and infusion rate. A note of this value should be made on the technical data sheet and is a useful reference at the reporting stage when considering attenuation and image quality issues.

Adenosine should be administered at a rate of $140\,\mu g/kg/min$ over 4–6 minutes by a continuous peripheral intravenous infusion for cardiac stress testing. Maximum coronary vasodilatation occurs within the first minute following the onset of the adenosine infusion and continues until the drug is stopped. Dipyridamole should be administered at $0.56\,mg/kg$ intravenously over a 4-minute period and may be given as a pump or hand injection.

Our current vasodilator protocol uses a 5-minute adenosine infusion rather than the 'standard 6-minute', but there is good evidence to support a shorter-duration infusion of 3 or 4 minutes, and both protocols have been found to be equally effective for the detection of CAD.[12,13] Shorter infusion times have the advantage of improving patient tolerance due to the reduction in frequency and duration of side-effects, as well as significant cost benefits. In the current financial climate of healthcare in the UK, the abbreviated protocol is likely to become more commonplace as there are significant savings to be made against the cost of this relatively expensive pharmacological stress agent.

Pre-calculating the infusion rates/dose required and presenting in a tabulated form for a range of weight values gives users an easy reference source and removes the need to calculate the dose on an individual patient basis (Table 4.10). This also reduces the risk of an inaccurate calculation and subsequent drug administration error. An infusion pump capable of delivering adenosine at rates up to $350\,ml/h$ is required, as it is impractical to administer the drug as a hand injection.

Your local procedures and paperwork should ensure that all calculations involving drug administrations are routinely counterchecked by a second person.

5. *Carry out a medical history check.* A check to ensure that the patient has been allocated to the correct protocol and that there are no recent medical problems or

Table 4.10 Adenosine infusion rates calculated for a range of patient weight values. The infusion is prepared from vials of adenosine at a concentration of 3 mg/ml in vials of 10 ml. For a 70-kg patient and a 5-minute infusion, a total of 16.5 ml is required (total adenosine dose = 49.5 mg)

Patient weight (kg)	Adenosine infusion rate (140 μg/kg/min)	
	ml/min	ml/h
45–49	2.1	126
50–54	2.3	138
55–59	2.6	156
60–64	2.8	168
65–69	3.0	180
70–74	3.3	198
75–79	3.5	210
80–84	3.8	228
85–89	4.0	240
90–94	4.2	252
95–99	4.4	264
100–104	4.7	282
105–109	4.9	294
110–114	5.1	306
115–119	5.4	324
120–124	5.6	336
125–129	5.8	348

contraindications to proceeding with the stress test confirms that the administration of a radiopharmaceutical is justified. The administration of adenosine in actively asthmatic patients may cause bronchoconstriction and bronchospasm, and should therefore be avoided. Proceed with caution, or seek medical advice if there is a history of chronic obstructive pulmonary disease or well-controlled asthma, as previously discussed. Adenosine (and dipyridamole) have the potential to cause first-, second- or third-degree AV block, or sinus bradycardia due to a direct depressant effect on the SA and AV nodes, and is contraindicated in patients with a history of second-degree or higher AV block without a functioning pacemaker. Adenosine can be given in the presence of first-degree heart block, although caution should be exercised, as a proportion of patients may progress to a higher degree of block.

6. *Give a detailed explanation of the procedure given and obtain consent.* A detailed explanation of the procedure should always be given, outlining possible side-effects and complications. Documented side-effects are quite numerous with both adenosine and dipyridamole (Table 4.11), and the more persistent and serious effects can be reversed by the administration of intravenous aminophylline (75–250 mg), preferably no earlier than at least 3 minutes following the tracer injection. This is seldom required with adenosine due to the very short half-life (less than 10 seconds) so that

Table 4.11   Common side-effects following the administration of adenosine and dipyridamole

Adenosine: Side-effects are frequent (80% of patients) but usually self-limiting and short acting. It may be necessary to discontinue the infusion if side-effects become serious or intolerable

Dipyridamole: Over 50% of patients develop side-effects; however, the frequency is less than that observed with adenosine, but the duration is longer (20–40 min)

Most commonly: Flushing, chest pain, headache, dyspnoea and the urge to breathe deeply, dizziness, light headedness, chest pressure, discomfort in stomach, neck, throat or jaw

Chest pain is generally non-specific, not associated with any ECG changes, and therefore not necessarily indicative of coronary artery disease

Less frequently: Bronchospasm, hypotension, AV block, ST segment depression, arrhythmia, sweating, nasal congestion, nipple discomfort, nervousness, paraesthesia, tremors, drowsiness, tinnitus, blurred vision, dry mouth, metallic taste, discomfort in the leg, arm or back, weakness or urinary urgency

Early termination of adenosine infusion:

AV block: If sustained second- or third-degree AV block develops, the infusion should be stopped immediately. (If first-degree AV block occurs, the patient should be observed carefully, as a quarter of patients will progress to a higher degree of block)

Severe hypotension: Systolic BP < 80 mmHg

Wheezing

ST depression: > 2 mm or more associated with severe chest pain

---

any effects should disappear within seconds of terminating the infusion. However, it can be a more frequent occurrence with dipyridamole, where the vasodilator effects may last between 20 and 40 minutes following administration. Aminophylline should always be prescribed and administered by a clinician.

As before, all relevant information should be noted on the technical data sheet. A check of the pregnancy status of female patients of child-bearing age should be made, and a signature obtained on a disclosure form in line with local procedures. Verbal or written consent should be obtained as dictated by local policy.

Mechanism and protocol (Table 4.12)

Adenosine is a naturally occurring and direct-acting coronary vasodilator which plays an important part in the regulation of coronary flow. It directly stimulates the A2 purine receptors, which causes coronary vasodilatation (increased flow) as well as systemic vasodilatation (decrease in blood pressure). The non-selective activation of A1, A2b, and A3 receptors causes many of the undesirable side-effects associated with an adenosine infusion: A1 purine receptors in the SA and AV node, which can lead to AV conduction delays and slowing of the heart rate; peripheral vasodilatation (A2b receptor); and bronchospasm (A2b and A3 receptors).

Table 4.12   Adenosine protocol (5-minute infusion)

- Record a baseline BP, HR and standard 12-lead ECG. Look for evidence of heart block on the ECG (note the PR interval). Abnormal findings of any of the baseline values will necessitate a reevaluation of the stress protocol. The BP should be measured in the arm opposite the adenosine infusion to avoid an adenosine bolus effect

- Insert two cannulas (one in each arm where possible) to avoid interrupting the adenosine infusion during administration of the activity and reduce risk of a bolus of adenosine when the tracer is administered. For a single cannula, use with a three-way tap to minimise interruption of adenosine during tracer administration and closely monitor patient for signs of a bolus effect

- Draw up the required amount of adenosine (plus 1.0 ml extra to allow for wastage in the infusion line). Perform a second-person check of the drug vials for contents and expiry date, and the dose administration rate

- Administer adenosine infusion at 140 μg/kg/min for 5 minutes

- During the infusion, record BP and HR, and obtain 12-lead ECG at 2 and 4 minutes, and at 2 minutes after the end of the infusion. Maintain constant observation of the ECG display during infusion

- Inject radiopharmaceutical after 3 minutes of adenosine infusion

- If first-degree AV block occurs – continue with the infusion and monitor very closely

- If second- or third-degree block occurs – discontinue adenosine infusion immediately. The AV block should resolve spontaneously within 15–30 seconds. If this does not happen – summon medical assistance immediately

- Continue to monitor ECG, BP and HR parameters following the end of infusion until any symptoms or side-effects alleviate

Following the administration of exogenous adenosine, a four- to five-fold increase in myocardial blood flow can be observed compared to the baseline resting blood flow (coronary flow reserve) in normal coronary vessels. In the presence of a significant coronary stenosis with reduced coronary flow reserve, the action of adenosine is attenuated as the vessel is unable to dilate further in response to pharmacological stimulation, resulting in heterogeneity of uptake following administration of a radioactive tracer.

Generally speaking the action of adenosine is not to compromise coronary flow, as seen with dynamic stress testing, but to accentuate the difference in myocardial blood flow between stenotic and normal vessels. This is then manifested as an overall increase in the uptake of radioactive tracer compared to resting baseline levels. However, in certain circumstances adenosine can cause a decrease in coronary blood flow in a stenosed vessel, resulting in myocardial ischaemia which may be associated with typical anginal symptoms and ECG changes. This is due to the development of 'coronary steal'.

Coronary steal is a phenomenon whereby the region of myocardium supplied by a severely stenosed coronary artery is also dependent upon collateral vessels which arise from remote arteries. Blood flow through the collaterals is reliant on perfusion pressure which can fall, particularly if they are supplied by a vessel containing a moderate stenosis. Thus, in this instance the administration of adenosine reduces collateral flow, and flow to the myocardium supplied by the severely stenosed vessel may reduce compared to the resting state. The resulting hypoperfusion may then cause true myocardial ischaemia. The development of severe ECG changes during adenosine stress testing (as demonstrated in Figure 4.2) indicative of widespread ischaemia should always be promptly communicated to the referring cardiologist (especially if associated with symptoms), as the patient may require urgent coronary angiography and intervention.

Dipyridamole was the first pharmacological stress agent to be introduced in the 1980s and is an indirect coronary artery vasodilator. It inhibits the intracellular reabsorption of endogenous adenosine, which leads to an increase in the amount of extracellular adenosine available to stimulate the purine receptors, leading to relaxation of vascular smooth muscle and subsequent increased blood flow due to coronary vasodilatation.

Dipyridamole should be infused at a dose rate of 0.56 mg/kg intravenously over 4 minutes and administered by hand injection or infusion pump. A pump is the preferred option as it is important to ensure that the drug is delivered slowly. Increasing the volume in the syringe by the addition of normal saline makes this an easier process for either hand or pump injection. The tracer is injected between 3 and 5 minutes after completion of the dipyridamole infusion (Figure 4.3).

COMBINED PHARMACOLOGICAL AND LOW-LEVEL EXERCISE PROTOCOL

Many departments now favour a combined exercise–adenosine stress method. This is an attractive technique for both patient and operator, as the combination of a vasodilator and physical stress results in a reduction of the severity and frequency of the unfavourable side-effects associated with adenosine stress alone. In addition, this method can result in enhancement of the image quality, although this is most likely a perceived effect due to the improved target to background ratio. As yet there is insufficient evidence to prove that the combined technique can lead to greater sensitivity for the detection of ischaemia in patients with coronary artery disease compared to adenosine alone;[14] however, there is evidence of increased detection of myocardial ischaemia using this technique, compared to MPS with a submaximal treadmill stress test.[15]

The decision to combine physical and pharmacological stress should be made on an individual patient basis by an experienced member of staff. There should be a high degree of confidence that there are no risks to the patient, particularly if they have failed to meet the criteria required for treadmill testing alone. The level of stress required for a combined study is generally considerably less than expected for a standard treadmill or bicycle protocol, and should be tailored to the physical ability of the

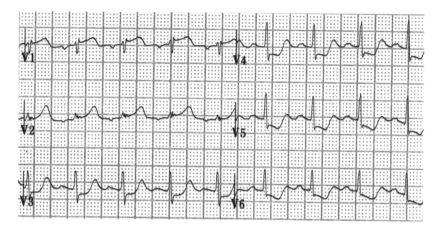

Figure 4.2   ECG demonstrating widespread ST and T-wave changes across all precordial chest leads 30 seconds after initiating the adenosine infusion. This degree of severity is indicative of severe coronary disease (see Chapter 7).

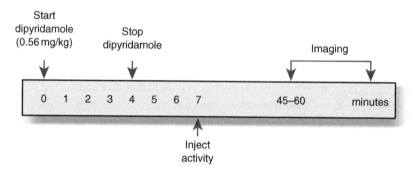

Figure 4.3   Dipyridamole stress protocol with imaging commencing between 45 and 60 minutes following tracer injection. Imaging up to 90 or 120 minutes post-injection may be necessary with delayed hepatobiliary clearance.

patient. This could involve the use of a different stress protocol, such as modified Bruce or Naughton, or simply 'holding' the treadmill on Stage 1 of the Bruce protocol (1.7 mph, 10% gradient), which is probably well within the physical capability of most patients. Combined studies can be performed on either an erect or supine bicycle ergometer if a treadmill is not available. As with other stress methods which induce an increase in heart rate, the use of low-level exercise combined with pharmacological stress is not recommended for patients with left bundle branch block or ventricular paced rhythm.

The same patient preparation and cardiac monitoring as for the adenosine protocol should be followed. It is not necessary to stop any rate limiting drugs prior to a combined protocol, as it is not important to achieve a target predicted heart rate. In a typical protocol the exercise duration is 6 minutes and the adenosine infusion is started after 1 minute and administered over 4 minutes. The activity is injected at 3 minutes (Figure 4.4).

Using a combined dipyridamole and treadmill or bicycle exercise method is also an option, and has been a recognised procedure since the early 1990s. Again, the benefits of combining vasodilator stress with low-level exercise are a significant reduction in the number of side-effects and improved image quality. The dipyridamole is administered as before (0.56 mg/kg over 4 minutes), and low-level exercise follows immediately after for a period of 6 minutes. The activity is injected after 3 minutes of exercise (Figure 4.5).

DOBUTAMINE STRESS PROCEDURE

Patient preparation

The same preparation for treadmill testing can be applied to dobutamine stress, but it is not necessary to discontinue aminophylline, theophylline, caffeine and other methylxanthines as the patient will not be receiving adenosine. The same exclusion criteria for treadmill testing also apply to dobutamine stress, other than the physical inability to exercise (Figure 4.4).

Care should be taken when administering dobutamine to patients with a history of ventricular arrhythmias or recent myocardial infarction as there is an increased risk of developing further complex arrhythmias with higher dose rates.

Weigh patient and calculate dobutamine dose and infusion rate. Weigh the patient to calculate the radiopharmaceutical dose required and to determine the dobutamine dose and infusion rate (ml/h). As before, a note of this value should be made on the technical data sheet, and is a useful reference at the reporting stage when considering attenuation and image quality issues.

Dobutamine is administered via an infusion pump in 3-minute stages at typical incremental doses of 5, 10, 15, 20, 30 and 40 µg/kg/min, and is supplied in 20-ml vials containing 250 mg of dobutamine. Before use, the vial needs to be diluted to a volume of 50 ml in a syringe for ease of administration. You may be able to obtain dobutamine from your pharmacy already diluted in syringes; however, this does shorten the shelf-life of the drug. Diluted dobutamine needs to be kept refrigerated, and you need to place individual orders for scheduled patients. If you are able to store dobutamine in your drug cupboard in the department, then it is a simple enough task to prepare a vial for a stress patient:

- Dilute a 20-ml (250 mg) vial of dobutamine to 50 ml in a syringe with 0.09% sodium chloride – concentration is now 5 mg/ml.
- Initial infusion rate (5 µg/kg/min) in ml/h can then be calculated as patient weight (kg) × 0.06.

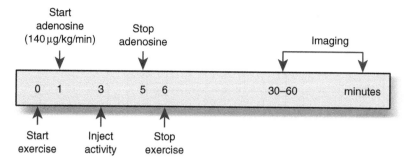

Figure 4.4 A combined adenosine and low-level exercise protocol, with imaging commencing between 30 and 60 minutes following tracer injection. Imaging up to 90 or 120 minutes post-injection may be necessary with delayed hepatobiliary clearance.

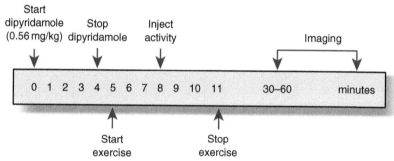

Figure 4.5 A combined dipyridamole and low-level exercise protocol with imaging commencing between 30 and 60 minutes following tracer injection. Imaging up to 90 or 120 minutes post-injection may be necessary with delayed hepatobiliary clearance.

Example:

- patient weight $= 70\,kg$
- initial rate of $5\,\mu g/kg/min = 70 \times 0.06 = 4.2\,ml/h$
- therefore incremental doses are: 4.2; 8.4; 12.6; 16.8; 25.2; and 33.6 ml/h.

The appropriate calculations can be entered on to a database or stress record sheet (Table 4.13). Any calculations involving the administration of drugs to patients should always be checked and countersigned by a second person to minimise the risk of drug administration errors. Your local protocols and procedures should specify this as an essential requirement.

MECHANISM AND PROTOCOL (TABLE 4.14)

Dobutamine is a potent synthetic catecholamine which has both strong positive inotropic and chronotropic effects. The respective effects are an increase in the

Table 4.13 Example of a record sheet for a dobutamine stress protocol

Dobutamine myocardial perfusion imaging

Name:
DOB:
Hospital no:
Weight:
Date:

Infusion rate (kg/min)	ml/h	Duration (min)	Heart rate	BP	Rate pressure product	Anginal score (1–10)	ECG changes	Symptoms/comments
Pre-test								
5 µg								
10 µg								
15 µg								
20 µg								
25 µg								
30 µg								
35 µg								
40 µg								
Recovery 3 min								
Recovery 10 min								

Dobutamine dose: Dilute 1 vial of dobutamine hydrochloride to 50 ml with saline.
Initial infusion rate (ml/h) = **Patient wt (kg) ×0.06** (5 µg/kg/min dose rate)

Dobutamine batch no: Expiry: Supervised by:

Table 4.14   Dobutamine protocol

- Record a baseline 12-lead ECG and repeat at the end of each 3-minute dose increment throughout the test. Maintain observation of real-time ECG display to monitor ST segment and T-wave changes and detect arrhythmias

- Record a baseline blood pressure (BP) and heart rate (HR) and repeat at the end of each dose increment. Abnormal findings of any of the baseline values (ECG, BP and HR) will necessitate a reevaluation of the stress protocol

- Calculate the baseline rate pressure product (RPP) and repeat at the end of each 3-minute stage and record:
  RPP = systolic pressure × heart rate

- Insert IV cannula – arm opposite the BP cuff – and flush with sodium chloride 0.9% injection to ensure patency. Attach an extension with a three-way connector to aid the injection and minimise the risk of a spill during administration of activity

- Prepare dobutamine infusion (250 mg dobutamine in 50 ml) and calculate dose rate. Perform a second-person check of the drug vial for contents and expiry date, and the dose administration rate

- Start infusion at 5 µg/kg/min and increase at 3-minute intervals to 10, 15, 20, 30 and 40 µg/kg/min

- Administer IV atropine (300–600 µg) if there has been inadequate heart rate response at maximum infusion rate or start hand-grip exercise (see text)

- Inject radiopharmaceutical at 85% MPHR or when maximum infusion rate is achieved and continue with the infusion for 1–2 minutes post-injection (refer to Chapter 5 for dose schedule)

- Continue to monitor ECG, BP and HR parameters during recovery until they return close to baseline, or until any ischaemic changes recover

- Record the exercise duration, symptoms, ECG changes and reason for stopping the test

contractility and cardiac output of the heart at lower doses, and an increase in the heart rate at higher infusion levels. Like physical exercise, dobutamine increases the myocardial oxygen demand and so increases regional myocardial blood flow. Robinson[16] postulated in 1967 that the heart rate and systolic pressure were probably the most important variables determining changes in myocardial oxygen consumption between rest and exercise, and first used the rate pressure product as an index of myocardial work. The rate pressure product (RPP) is the product of heart rate (HR) multiplied by systolic pressure (SP). As contractility is an important factor contributing to myocardial oxygen consumption, the RPP is a useful indicator of the level of stress achieved during dobutamine stress testing. As a general guideline, we would be happy with a minimum of a two-fold increase in the RPP from baseline to peak stress during a dobutamine infusion.

The single most difficult part of performing a dobutamine stress test is determining the point of peak stress and, therefore, the most appropriate time to inject the radiopharmaceutical. Patients do not respond physiologically to a pharmacological stimulus in the same way that they respond to a physical challenge, and there is a huge variation in response between individuals. Many clinical protocols and procedure guidelines use the same endpoint for injecting the radiopharmaceutical during dobutamine stress as for treadmill testing – 85% MPHR – but it can be very difficult to achieve this target using dobutamine stress alone, due to other physiological responses. With increasing heart rate, a mismatch develops between cardiac output and the venous return due to physical inactivity, and this increases the potential for vasovagal syncope at higher dose rates. It is important therefore to watch the patient closely during the infusion to determine whether they reach a 'plateau' stage where further increases of the dose do not result in further increases in the heart rate. At this point there is the option to administer intravenous atropine to give the heart rate another push towards 85% MPHR; however, we favour the use of moderate exercise in the form of hand-grips during peak stress. Fortunately this is not a problem that we encounter too frequently, as we perform limited numbers of dobutamine studies since moving to adenosine as our primary stress agent of choice.

REFERENCES

1. Statutory Instrument 2000 No 1059. The Ionising Radiation (Medical Exposure) Regulations 2000. London: The Stationery Office, 2000. (online at http://www.opsi.gov.uk)
2. Department of Health. Toolkit for producing patient information. Version 2.0, 2003. (online at http://www.nhsidentity.nhs.uk/)
3. Levine MG, Ahlberg AW, Mann A et al. Comparison of exercise, dipyridamole, adenosine, and dobutamine stress with the use of Tc-99m tetrofosmin tomographic imaging. J Nucl Cardiol 1999; 4: 389–96.
4. The Royal College of Radiologists. Skills Mix in Clinical Radiology. London: The Royal College of Radiologists, 1999. (online at http://www.rcr.ac.uk)
5. Tahir T, Gutierrez R. Comparing stress testing methods: available techniques and their use in CAD evaluation. Postgrad Med 2004; 115: 61–70.
6. Underwood SR, Anagnostopoulos C, Cerqueira C et al. Myocardial perfusion scintigraphy: the evidence. Eur J Nucl Med Mol Imaging 2004; 31: 261–91.
7. Hansen CL. The conundrum of left bundle branch block. J Nucl Cardiol 2004; 1: 90–2.
8. Reyes E, Loong CY, Latus K, Anagnostopoulos C, Underwood SR. Safety and tolerability of adenosine stress MPI in patients with asthma or chronic obstructive airways disease. J Nucl Cardiol 2004; 11: S5 (abstr).
9. Samady H, Wackers FJ, Joska TM, Zaret BL, Jain D. Pharmacologic stress perfusion imaging with adenosine: role of simultaneous low-level treadmill exercise. J Nucl Cardiol 2002; 9: 188–96.
10. Gruning T, Brogsitter C, Khonsari M et al. Can administration of metoclopramide reduce artefacts related to abdominal activity in myocardial perfusion SPECT? Nucl Med Commun 2006; 27: 953–7.
11. Nesto RW, Kowalchuk GJ. The ischemic cascade: temporal sequence of hemodynamic, electrocardiographic and symptomatic expressions of ischemia. Am J Cardiol 1987; 59: 23C–30C.
12. O'Keefe JH Jr, Bateman TM, Handlin LR, Barnhart CS. Four- versus 6-minute infusion protocol for adenosine thallium-201 single photon emission computed tomography imaging. Am Heart J 1995; 129: 482–7.

13. Treuth MG, Reyes GA, He ZX et al. Tolerance and diagnostic accuracy of an abbreviated adenosine infusion for myocardial scintigraphy: a randomized, prospective study. J Nucl Cardiol 2001; 8: 548–54.

14. Jamil G, Ahlberg AW, Elliott MD et al. Impact of limited treadmill exercise on adenosine Tc-99m sestamibi single-photon emission computed tomographic myocardial perfusion imaging in coronary artery disease. Am J Cardiol 1999; 84: 400–3.

15. Holly TA, Satran A, Bromet DS et al. The impact of adjunctive adenosine infusion during exercise myocardial perfusion imaging: results of the Both Exercise and Adenosine Stress Test (BEAST) trial. J Nucl Cardiol 2003; 10: 291–6.

16. Robinson BF. Relation of heart rate and systolic blood pressure to the onset of pain in angina pectoris. Circulation 1967; 35: 1073–83.

5

Scanning the patient

Scanning of the patient is arguably the most critical stage in the whole myocardial perfusion scintigraphy (MPS) process, since the entire study will have been a waste of time if the images produced are not of the highest quality. Single photon emission computed tomography (SPECT) imaging is the least tolerant of all nuclear medicine techniques when it comes to allowing for poor quality scans due to patient size, movement or inadequate count statistics, and nowhere is this more true than in cardiac SPECT imaging. Cardiac contraction and respiration already have a significant influence upon the degradation of image resolution, so any patient movement in either a vertical or a horizontal plane will result in further impairment as well as introduce image artefacts at the reconstruction stage (see Chapter 6).

It is assumed that the reader will undertake SPECT imaging only (rather than planar imaging), and due to the poor imaging characteristics of thallium in SPECT imaging, the remainder of this chapter deals entirely with techniques using the technetium agents tetrofosmin and sestamibi.

RADIOPHARMACEUTICAL DOSE

The Administration of Radioactive Substances Advisory Committee (ARSAC)[1] guidance recommends diagnostic reference levels (DRLs) for SPECT imaging using the technetium agents as follows:

- **1-day protocol:** total of 1000 MBq (250 MBq for first scan and 750 MBq for second scan)
- **2-day protocol:** 400 MBq for each study.

The Ionising Radiation (Medical Exposure) Regulations 2000[2] define DRLs as:

'dose levels in medical radiodiagnostic practices or, in the case of radioactive medicinal products, levels of activity, for typical examinations for groups of standard sized patients or standard phantoms for broadly defined types of equipment'.

This is the premise under which ARSAC have established DRLs, and they do not expect these levels to be exceeded for standard procedures when applying principles of good practice in the UK. ARSAC does accept, however, that it may be necessary to exceed the recommended activities in individual patients where clinical circumstances make it necessary. This tends to be a relatively frequent occurrence in the client group that are referred for cardiac imaging.

A good proportion of patients referred for myocardial perfusion imaging are 'overweight', which is hardly surprising as obesity is a significant risk factor for coronary disease. Increasing the acquisition time for SPECT imaging can compensate for the low count rate in this group of patients, but it is often problematic as there is an increased probability of movement artefact. Younger and fitter patients are capable of tolerating lengthy imaging times, but this can be too difficult for the older patient group, especially where there are additional medical problems or disabilities present, such as arthritis. It is therefore important to ensure that patient size and physical capability are assessed on arrival in the department, in order to establish the dose required on an individual patient basis.

In our department, both weight and height are taken into consideration when assessing patient size, as well as breast size in female patients.

Using the 2-day protocol, patients are given a standard 400-MBq dose up to 90 kg weight in males and 85 kg weight in females for stress imaging. Above these values, the dose is calculated at 5 MBq per kg of body weight to a maximum value of 600 MBq.

For rest imaging with gated SPECT, the standard minimum dose is 500 MBq for all patients, and the dose calculated at 5 MBq per kg of body weight above 100 kg up to a maximum of 600 MBq.

A 'visual' size assessment is currently used to amend these values if the patient is exceptionally short or tall in stature. Occasionally this may also result in a decrease in the standard dose where the patient is smaller than an average size patient. We are currently looking at calculating the dose required relative to other indicators of patient size such as the body mass index (BMI) and waist measurements, which should remove the need to perform a subjective visual assessment of the body habitus. The increased DRL for gated SPECT imaging is justified, as it is accepted that more counts are required to produce high quality studies with relatively short imaging times. Administering standard 400-MBq doses for gated SPECT studies is therefore likely to result in a substandard investigation, and either an equivocal result or a requirement for repeat imaging resulting in an even greater radiation exposure to the patient.

It is also possible to administer an increased dose for patients who are likely to pose particular problems with attenuation when using a 1-day protocol, but the recommendation is to maintain a ratio of at least 3:1 between the first and second doses and a minimum 2-hour delay between the stress and rest images. Many departments now perform a single-day protocol without a delay between the stress and rest injections, but this requires an increase in the dose ratio to between 3.5:1 and 4:1 to maintain the count density ratio between the studies.[3] This would result in doses which would be prohibitive in some patients, and so in those cases, a 2-day imaging protocol is preferable.

Table 5.1   Comparison of 1-day and 2-day protocols for myocardial perfusion scintigraphy

1-day protocol

- The investigation can be completed on one hospital visit, but is a lengthy appointment

- May require a time delay up to 2–3 hours between rest and stress injections

- The extent and severity of perfusion defects may be underestimated when using a rest–stress technique due to cross-talk of activity from the rest injection

- Resting perfusion may not be optimal if the patient has stopped taking antianginal medication

- Left ventricular (LV) ejection fraction obtained with gated SPECT if performed after stress may not reflect a true resting measurement (due to post-stress stunning)

- Not a suitable technique for overweight patients due to low dose administered for the first study

2-day protocol

- Reduced appointment length but requires two hospital visits

- No cross-talk of activity between stress and rest imaging

- Resting perfusion can be optimised as the patient can continue taking antianginal medication

- Gated SPECT can be performed during rest study with improved accuracy of assessment of LV function

- Can administer an increased dose for overweight patients

IMAGING PROTOCOLS

As implied above, MPS can be performed using either a 1-day or a 2-day protocol, and there are distinct advantages and disadvantages to using either technique from qualitative, technical and scheduling points of view (Table 5.1). The choice will be dependent upon the service that you are able to provide as well as the resources available. From a clinical perspective, the 1-day and 2-day protocols have been compared using the technetium agents and found to produce comparable results.[4,5]

1-day protocol

As the name implies, both stress and rest studies are performed on the same day. Many departments advocate the use of this protocol, and generally refer to the convenience of a single visit to the hospital for the patient as a major advantage. The rest–stress strategy is generally preferred to stress–rest for the 1-day protocol, as the images obtained from a rest study following a stress study may demonstrate incomplete or little 'reversibility'. This may be due to the inhomogeneity of the background caused by defects on the stress images which persist on the delayed rest images, or may be due to perfusion abnormalities which persist following an episode of transient stress-induced myocardial ischaemia after normal flow has been restored in the coronary artery.[6] These scenarios will result in a report that significantly underestimates the degree of reversibility and will have consequences for the future clinical management of the patient.

2-day protocol

Stress and rest imaging is performed on two separate days which need not be consecutive. The time delay ensures that the second study is not contaminated by any residual activity from the first study. Many departments who only perform cardiac imaging on 1 day per week have a schedule whereby the stress imaging is performed in the morning and the rest imaging is performed in the afternoon of the same day of the following week.

Performing the rest study on a different day from the stress test will result in improved image quality through elimination of the stress background activity. In addition, the patient can remain on all antianginal medication for the rest study, which maximises the potential resting perfusion and subsequent tracer uptake.

Our department routinely performs a 2-day protocol, which allows us to schedule the greatest number of tests per day. The studies are generally scheduled in no particular order for stress or rest. The only exceptions are in patients with known severe coronary artery disease, previous extensive myocardial infarction, or left ventricular failure, where the rest study is always scheduled first to enable an assessment of resting perfusion and left ventricular function to be made prior to performing a stress test. If either perfusion or function is found to be significantly impaired at this stage, the images are reviewed with the reporting clinician or referring cardiologist (Figure 5.1). A decision on whether or not to proceed can then be made based on the risk of compromising perfusion and function further following stress testing.

Acute referrals and requests for inpatient scans can be slotted into the schedule relatively easily as a single-day protocol if necessary, by performing the studies at the beginning of the morning session and end of the afternoon session, and provision can be made within the appointment template to accommodate such referrals.

Stress-only imaging

Performing the stress imaging first offers the potential advantage of being able to cancel the rest scan if normal perfusion has been demonstrated on the stress images. Not only is there a significant reduction in the radiation exposure to the patient, but also this represents a more efficient way of working, with consequent cost benefits. This is a good theoretical model, but from a practical perspective there are several problems with the approach, particularly if you are using the single-day

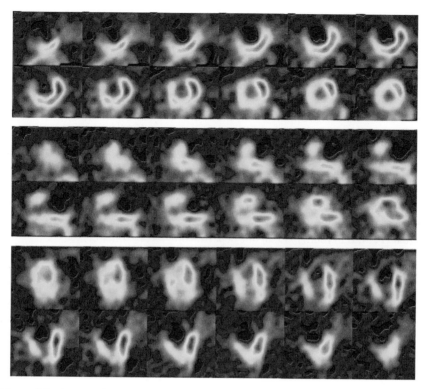

Figure 5.1 A rest-only study demonstrating a large perfusion defect involving the anterior wall and septum. Gated imaging demonstrated impaired left ventricular function (ejection fraction calculated at 29%) with a dyskinetic apex indicating the presence of an aneurysm. The images were reviewed with the cardiologist and the stress study was cancelled.

protocol. The 1-day protocol DRL recommends a split of 250–750 MBq for the dose administration. The stress imaging would therefore need to be performed using only 250 MBq of activity, resulting in longer imaging times with an increased possibility of patient movement. In the event of motion-induced image artefacts, this would clearly make it more difficult for the reporting clinician to interpret the scan as normal. In addition, it is not best practice to perform gated imaging on the 1-day stress study due to the low count rate.

There is also a school of thought that balanced three-vessel coronary disease may produce the same appearance as a normal scan.[7] The interpretation of SPECT perfusion images is dependent upon the relative regional distribution of activity in the myocardium, and balanced coronary disease can present as a uniform distribution. Quantification of tracer uptake in the myocardium is necessary and highly valuable in this patient group to distinguish normal from impaired myocardial perfusion, which requires reference to both stress and rest images (see Chapter 6).

Performing a 2-day protocol will also allow you to cancel the resting study following a 'normal' stress perfusion scan, but with the added bonus of administering a larger patient dose with a subsequent improvement in image quality. However, the possibility of missing balanced three-vessel disease still remains a concern.

REST IMAGING AND NITRATES

There is good evidence to support the routine use of glyceryl trinitrate (GTN) prior to the rest injection.[8,9] GTN dilates blood vessels and increases the supply of blood and oxygen to the heart while reducing its workload, and given 1–2 minutes before the resting injection can increase the radiopharmaceutical uptake leading to enhanced detection of viable myocardium. This technique, using two puffs of sublingual GTN, is in routine use in our department.

It is essential to ascertain whether your patient has already been prescribed GTN and the frequency with which they use it. GTN can cause severe headaches as well as severe hypotension and bradycardia. These side-effects are more common in first-time users of GTN, which should therefore be withheld in this group of patients unless medical support is readily available.

IMAGE ACQUISITION

There is a considerable difference in opinion about the optimum imaging times following administration of the activity. Generally longer delays between injection and acquisition are required for the resting images, and also the stress images using pharmacological stimulation compared to treadmill stress studies. As previously discussed in Chapter 2, there are discernible differences in hepatobiliary clearance rates between sestamibi and tetrofosmin (Figure 5.2), and this will determine the most favourable imaging times. Scanning the patient too early following the tracer injection will most likely result in potentially uninterpretable defects in the inferior wall, especially where the concentration of the subdiaphragmatic activity is greater than or equal to the concentration of activity within the myocardium.

Whichever imaging agent you select for use in your department, imaging should only commence after the hepatobiliary activity has sufficiently cleared. Locally developed imaging protocols should indicate acceptable times to commence imaging following injection for both the stress and rest studies, but it should be noted that there will be considerable variation between patients, and an assessment of image quality should always be made prior to commencing the SPECT or gated study. This may simply be a visual evaluation of the persistence image, or possibly acquisition of a single planar image using an anterior or left anterior oblique (LAO) projection which the operator may find useful.

Imaging with tetrofosmin can usually begin 15–30 minutes following a treadmill stress injection, and 45–60 minutes after a rest injection or pharmacological stress.

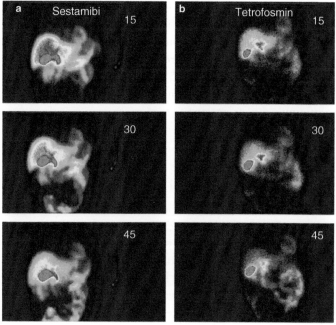

Figure 5.2 Planar rest images from two patients, using sestamibi (a) and tetrofosmin (b). Top row is 15 minutes post-injection, then 30 and 45 minutes are below. Although there is clearly likely to be considerable variation in hepatobiliary clearance between patients, these images are fairly representative of the results using these radiopharmaceuticals. Note the higher levels of hepatobiliary and gut activity with Sestamibi.

For sestamibi the imaging times should be increased to 30 minutes post treadmill exercise and 90–120 minutes following injection at rest or pharmacological stress.

Selection of optimum scanning times is likely to be linked to the work schedule in the department as well as the agent in routine use. It should be stressed, however, that regardless of the imaging sequence used, all images must be assessed for quality (see below) before the patient leaves the department. All cardiac software allows the user to reconstruct the slice images fairly rapidly, so it is a simple process to inspect them visually for evidence of substantial subdiaphragmatic activity before sending the patient home. Substandard images should always be repeated, and there are very few exceptional circumstances where repeat imaging should be waived.

Our patients are routinely starved for 4 hours prior to both stress and rest appointments and are encouraged to eat following the injection. Theoretically this aids clearance of tracer from the liver and gall bladder, although there is no definitive evidence to support this. In some patients eating may be counterproductive if there is retrograde movement of activity from the duodenum to the stomach, or if the tracer reaches the transverse colon too quickly, although our experience has shown that this will occur in some patients whether they have eaten or not (for example, those with a history of hiatus hernia, incompetent pyloric sphincter or gastro-oesophageal reflux). As discussed in Chapter 4, metoclopramide should be given to promote gastric emptying in patients with high levels of activity within the stomach, or prior to the tracer injection for the second scan if the first scan had demonstrated marked gastric activity. Other methods to help reduce the amount of activity within the stomach include asking the patient to walk around between the injection and imaging, and drinking 2–3 glasses of cold water 15 minutes before imaging commences. We have found this to be a useful strategy, and it is a common practice in many establishments performing cardiac imaging.

PATIENT POSITIONING

The patient should be supine with both arms above the head where possible, and supported in a comfortable position. If there is a particular difficulty in maintaining both arms above the head for the entire duration of the scan, then it is possible to image the patient with the right arm down by the side (Figure 5.3).

It is far better to ensure that the patient is comfortable before imaging commences than to try and make adjustments half way through the scan – this most certainly will lead to artefacts on the resultant images. Knee support is also helpful, and should be used routinely during cardiac imaging, as patient comfort is crucial to minimise movement during the acquisition.

Imaging the patient in a prone position has been suggested to reduce the incidence of inferior attenuation artefacts, but it can be difficult to reproduce exactly the same position for both the stress and rest scans, and can produce an anteroseptal defect secondary to an increase in sternal attenuation. Prone imaging should only be used in combination with, and not as a replacement for, supine imaging, which leads to increased imaging times per patient.

Some procedure guidelines advocate that female patients should be imaged without a bra to minimise attenuation in the anterior wall. But depending upon the size and the density of the patient's breasts, this method is likely to introduce artefacts from attenuation in random areas of the myocardium due to the uncertain position of the breast during the image acquisition. The availability of gated SPECT and attenuation correction packages provides an alternative solution for assessing defects due to attenuation.

It is also possible to use a chest compression band to minimise breast attenuation; however, this method can potentially increase attenuation defects as it is entirely dependent upon how the band is applied. Consistency in positioning of the chest band is required between the stress and rest scans, or it may be difficult to distinguish defects from artefacts on the reconstructed images.

Female patients attending for MPS in our department are not asked to remove any of their underclothes, but we do ask them to wear the same bra on both visits to ensure that there is relatively good reproducibility of positioning when they return for the second scan. A note is made of the patient's bra size on the technical data sheet as an aid to interpretation at the reporting stage, as well as any other relevant information

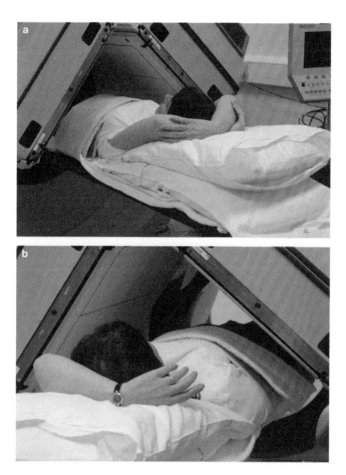

Figure 5.3 Good positioning for cardiac imaging with both arms raised above the head (a). Not all patients will be capable of achieving or maintaining this position for the duration of the scan so imaging with the right arm down by the side is also possible (b). A yellow immobilization band can be seen in place.

which may result in unusual appearances such as a previous mastectomy or insertion of breast implants.

We routinely use a chest band as a method of motion restriction during the image acquisition (Figure 5.3). The band is applied so that it provides support for the patient and aids in their level of comfort and feeling of security when lying on a narrow scanning bed. The band is not particularly tight when applied, and has been found to be successful in reducing motion-induced artefacts.

Most of the current equipment manufacturers provide support and restraint aids as standard features, particularly with dedicated cardiac systems, where the equipment has been designed to specifically address these issues in cardiac imaging. This is clearly evident when comparing the two gamma cameras in Figures 5.3 and 5.4.

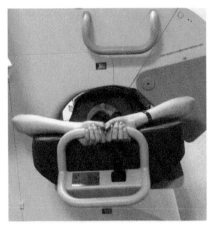

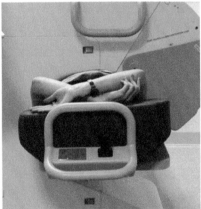

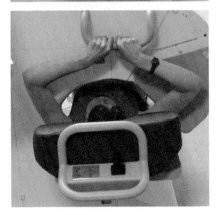

Figure 5.4 A dedicated cardiac gamma camera with a range of hand-grips. This provides a number of different options for arm positioning, and it is usually possible to find one that is comfortable for the patient. It is important to tell them not to change their position during scanning.

Older equipment or general purpose gamma cameras may need to be adapted, or additional accessories purchased to ensure that patient movement is kept to a minimum during cardiac imaging.

Making sure that your patient understands how the imaging will be performed, the length of time it is likely to take, and what is expected of them is vital before the imaging commences. We stress the importance of remaining as still as possible, and ask our patients to refrain from talking once the acquisition has started, unless they have any real concerns or problems. Ambient music and lighting can help to create an atmosphere that is calm and relaxing, but try not to overdo it, or your patient may drift off to sleep. Patients who fall asleep during the acquisition may have artefacts on the reconstructed images due to a gradual change in the position of the heart as the body relaxes; and sleeping during gated imaging will probably result in a drop in heart rate below the window of accepted beats (see below – 'Gated SPECT imaging'). Regular updates about the progress of the scan from the operator should encourage the patient to stay awake, as long as they have been instructed not to respond to your commentary. Be wary of waking the patient during the acquisition as they may awaken in a startled manner, and this will most certainly result in images degraded by movement artefact.

ACQUISITION PARAMETERS

- Image acquisition should only be performed using a gamma camera that has undergone regular quality control checks and has achieved the standards for SPECT acquisition as determined by local policy and procedures.
- High resolution collimators are recommended.
- A standard 15–20% energy window centred at 140 keV for technetium-99m-labelled radiopharmaceuticals should be selected.
- It is possible to use zoom during the acquisition, but it is not routinely recommended. It is fairly easy to miss the heart (typically the apex) from the field of view due to the difficulty of accurately assessing cardiac size from the persistence mode image. And while it is possible to do a 'trial-run' with the gamma cameras around the patient to check positioning across the entire acquisition arc, this will add considerably to the length of time that the patient has to lie on the scanning table. It is more appropriate to use a post-reconstruction software zoom, which should be standardised for all patient studies (see Chapter 6).

Make sure that all scanning parameters used during the first acquisition are written down on the technical data sheet to ensure reproduction for the second acquisition – particularly the height of the scanning table if this is a variable factor.

SINGLE PHOTON EMISSION COMPUTED TOMOGRAPHY IMAGING

Tomographic imaging with a single- or dual-head gamma camera is typically performed using a 180° rotation. It is also possible to acquire SPECT images using a 360° rotation, but a 180° acquisition is generally preferred due to improved resolution, shorter imaging times, and fewer problems with attenuation defects. The cameras obtain data from a 45° right anterior oblique (RAO) projection to a 45° left posterior oblique (LPO) projection.

With a dual-headed camera the heads are generally positioned at 90° to each other during a 180° rotation (Figure 5.5), with each head travelling through 90° using a circular or non-circular orbit as discussed in Chapter 2.

Images are acquired using a 'step-and-shoot' method, typically with 60–64 steps in the total acquisition depending on the starting position and the exact configuration of the camera heads. The detectors do not acquire any data as they move from one position to the next, which adds to the total imaging time. Some systems are capable of acquiring images in a continuous mode with improved image counts, but there is some loss of image resolution as a result of 'blurring', as the detectors continue to move at the same time as data are being acquired. The acquisition time at each step will depend upon the size of the patient and the activity administered. If you have adjusted the activity according to the patient's weight, then it is possible to use a fairly standard acquisition time for all patients, irrespective of their size. The aim should be to ensure that the total imaging time is kept below 30 minutes to minimise the risk of patient movement due to discomfort.

For a 90° dual-headed camera system acquiring 32 projections for each detector (64 images in total), the time per projection would be 25–30 seconds for 400–600 MBq of activity, with a total scan time of approximately 16–22 minutes. We use a 128 × 128 matrix size with zoom at the reconstruction stage (see Chapter 6), but a 64 × 64 matrix is perfectly acceptable for SPECT acquisitions.

For the 1-day protocol it is necessary to adjust the imaging times accordingly: 25–40 seconds for a 250-MBq stress acquisition, and 20–30 seconds for a non-gated 750-MBq rest acquisition, depending upon patient size. As previously stated, the 2-day imaging protocol is preferable in larger patients to avoid restrictive dose limits and consequently prolonged imaging times.

GATED SPECT IMAGING

Gating is a technique in which the data acquisition is triggered by a start pulse from the patient's electrocardiogram (ECG; the R wave) during imaging. For gated SPECT imaging, the technique allows the data to be collected in multiple time intervals or frames (typically 8 or 16) across the cardiac cycle for each angle during the acquisition. The protocol can be set up to acquire either a specific number of beats

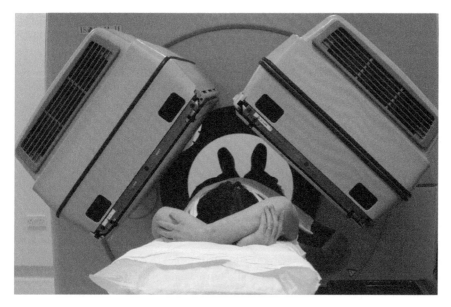

Figure 5.5 Large field of view (LFOV) dual-head gamma camera with the detectors moving to a 90° configuration for cardiac imaging.

per angle, or for a specific time interval per angle. Acquiring for a specified number of beats is preferred, as this method is more tolerant of gating errors due to arrhythmias than a timed acquisition when reconstructing the slices for functional analysis. This topic is discussed in more detail in Chapter 6.

As with SPECT imaging, you should aim to keep the total imaging time under 30 minutes to avoid problems with patient movement. As a general rule, the number of beats to acquire per angle should be half of the patient's heart rate in beats/min – this will ensure an acquisition time of at least 30 seconds per angle with a stable heart rate. We have found that this method will yield a good statistical result when imaging a patient following the administration of a weight-adjusted dose.

The beat window should be configured at around 20% to ensure that arrhythmias such as ventricular extrasystoles (VEs) are excluded during the acquisition. Inclusion of these data is possible if using a beat window that is too wide (>40%), which makes it difficult to assess the true end-systolic point during data reconstruction and quantification. The result will not be an accurate reflection of the left ventricular ejection fraction. An assessment of the beat histogram (if available) is a good method of assessing the quality of the investigation: you should expect to see a discrete peak centred in the beat window, whereas a histogram resembling a Gaussian distribution, or the presence of multiple peaks, is typical of poor quality gating.

Acquiring data over 16 frames rather than 8 will also result in improved accuracy when calculating the ejection fraction; however, this requires more counts to be obtained with increased imaging times.

Gated imaging can be performed following administration of activity at either stress or rest, but generally speaking is best performed on the rest study. The possibility of significant defects on the stress study means that the software would need to interpolate the edges of the myocardium during reconstruction of the gated data set, and due to the absence of counts in the defect, it may not always be particularly accurate. This can give the heart an unusual shape on the reconstructed images, make interpretation difficult, and reduce the accuracy of any left ventricular (LV) quantitative analysis (see Chapter 6). Unless the patient is being actively stressed at the time of the acquisition, the gated data represent the LV function at rest, irrespective of whether the activity was administered at stress or rest. However, an ischaemic episode during the stress test may take a considerable time to resolve in some patients (post-stress stunning), and the effects of this on the reconstructed gated images may include abnormalities of wall motion and thickness, increased LV volumes due to transient dilatation, and impaired LV ejection fraction. These abnormalities would not be apparent on gated imaging performed in the same patient following a rest injection. Therefore the best option would be to obtain gated data for both the stress and rest studies, as the presence of wall motion abnormalities and impaired LV function shown on imaging following a stress injection would be a clinically significant finding. Your choice to gate both studies, or a single study only (either stress or rest), is again a matter for local consideration. The argument against routinely gating both studies is the additional time that is needed to set up the patient prior to imaging. It should also be remembered that post-stress stunning is an intermittent and unpredictable occurrence, and so a lot of unhelpful stress gated acquisitions would result from a policy of routine rest and stress gating. The important issue is to decide on a protocol, and then stick to it. There is no value, and indeed it could be very misleading, if you hop from gating after stress to gating after rest injections in an extemporised fashion, and it will only confuse the reporting clinician.

As previously discussed, departments undertaking both stress and rest scans on the same day should perform gated SPECT on the second part of the study, whether stress or rest, in order to benefit from the substantially larger dose administered. It would be difficult, but not impossible, for the patient to tolerate the necessarily prolonged imaging time if gating was performed on the first part of the study.

The ECG electrodes should be attached to the patient's chest as soon as you have them lying on the scanning table (making sure that you do not overlay the heart with any metal studs or clips on the cable), and then allow at least 5 minutes for the heart rate to stabilise before starting the acquisition. During this time you can set up all the other parameters for the acquisition, and also remember to check the ECG display for gross arrhythmias, such as bigeminy, trigeminy or atrial fibrillation. The presence of an irregular heartbeat will not necessarily preclude you from performing gated imaging, but it will undoubtedly increase the scanning time (if acquiring for a specific number of beats per angle), and will most likely have a detrimental effect on the reconstruction of the perfusion slices from the summed gated data set.

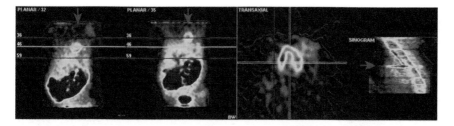

Figure 5.6   Movement artefact: the display shows planar frames 32 and 35 of a tomographic acquisition with the heart (arrows) moving out of the reconstruction boundaries on frame 35 – the vertical shift is well demonstrated on the sinogram (arrowed). The sinogram also shows evidence of poor gating with several 'low-count stripes' across the image.

Table 5.2   Summary of post-acquisition data quality checks for MPS SPECT and gated SPECT imaging using a dual-head gamma camera system

View the complete raw data set in a **cine display** (preferably following filtration) and process through to reconstruction of the standard slice data sets (see Chapter 6)

- **Are all the images present in the raw data set?** Check for blank or corrupted frames

- **Do all projections visually appear to have a similar count density?** Compare head 1 to head 2, and compare frames for a single detector

- **Is the transition of the images between the detectors smooth?** i.e. image 32 of head 1 and image 1 (33 in the series) of head 2

- **Is there evidence of patient movement in either a vertical or a horizontal plane?** Refer also to the sinogram image (Figure 5.6)

- **Is there adequate hepatobiliary clearance or evidence of other extracardiac activity?** The presence of a raised right hemidiaphragm can bring the gall bladder into close proximity with the left ventricle (Figure 5.7)

- **Any evidence of external attenuation defects?** e.g. electrodes, coins, etc.

- **Are there any sources of activity external to the chest which may impact upon reconstruction of the images?** e.g. injection site

- **Is the heart present on all images and not truncated at the apex?** Check that the heart does not drift off the field of view at the beginning and end of the data set

- **Is there evidence of 'flash' on the summed gated raw data set?** This would indicate a gating artefact possibly due to arrhythmias. Assess the heart rate histogram if available for a single discrete peak

A post-acquisition check of the summed gated data should always be performed to look for evidence of 'flash' on the planar images using a cine display, or 'stripes' across the sinogram (see below; Figure 5.6). If present, it will still be possible to use the reconstructed gated slices for functional analysis, but it will be necessary to repeat

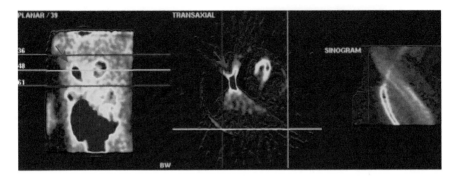

Figure 5.7   A patient with a raised hemidiaphragm on the right. The gall bladder is aligned with the heart seen on the planar and transaxial frames (arrows). The sinogram demonstrates the intensity of the activity in the gall bladder compared with the myocardial activity.

the acquisition without gating to produce the perfusion images (see Chapter 6 – 'Gating errors').

As with SPECT imaging, it is important to make sure that your patient is comfortable before starting the acquisition, not only to ensure that movement artefacts are kept to a minimum, but also because any discomfort may result in gating errors due to heart rate variability. Muscle spasm, pain and stress can all cause the heart rate to increase outside of the window for beat acceptance.

Post-acquisition check

Once the imaging is complete, you should perform a series of checks to establish the quality and precision of the acquired data before the patient is allowed to leave the department (Table 5.2; see Chapter 6). If the data fail to meet the expected standard, then the general rule should be for repeat imaging. It should be noted that it is not always possible to produce a set of images which completely satisfies your imaging standards criteria – some problems may be impossible to rectify.

A review of your imaging techniques or protocols should be undertaken if there are recurring imaging problems of a similar nature – for example high subdiaphragmatic uptake – indicating that imaging has commenced too early after administration of activity. An audit at the reporting stage can help to identify recurrent problems with image acquisition.

Some image problems may not be outwardly evident to the operator, and advice should be sought from a more experienced member of staff with advanced processing skills if there are any doubts about the quality of the acquired data. It is advisable to involve the person who will be processing the data through to the reporting stage, so that they can pass on any relevant information about the reconstructed data to the reporting clinician to aid with interpretation.

REFERENCES

1. Administration of Radioactive Substances Advisory Committee (ARSAC). Notes for Guidance on the Clinical Administration of Radiopharmaceuticals and Use of Sealed Radioactive Sources. Diagnostic Procedures – Adult Patients, March 2006: 33–8. (online at http://www.arsac.org.uk)
2. Statutory Instrument 2000 No 1059. The Ionising Radiation (Medical Exposure) Regulations 2000. London: The Stationery Office, 2000. (online at http://www.opsi.gov.uk)
3. Henzlova MJ, Cerqueira MD, Mahmarian JJ, Yao S. Stress protocols and tracers. J Nucl Cardiol 2006; 13: e80–90.
4. Taillefer R, Laflamme L, Dupras G et al. Myocardial perfusion imaging with 99mTc-methoxy-isobutyl-isonitrile (MIBI): comparison of short and long time intervals between rest and stress injections. Eur J Nucl Med 1988; 13: 515–22.
5. Borges-Neto S, Coleman RE, Jones RH. Perfusion and function at rest and treadmill exercise using technetium-99m-sestamibi: comparison of one- and two-day protocols in normal volunteers. J Nucl Med 1990; 31: 1128–32.
6. Fram DB, Azar RR, Ahlberg AW et al. Duration of abnormal SPECT myocardial perfusion imaging following resolution of acute ischemia: an angioplasty model. J Am Coll Cardiol 2003; 41: 452–9.
7. Aarnoudse WH, Botman KJ, Pijls NH. False-negative myocardial scintigraphy in balanced three-vessel disease, revealed by coronary pressure measurement. Int J Cardiovasc Intervent 2003; 5: 67–71.
8. Maurea S, Cuocolo A, Soricelli A et al. Enhanced detection of viable myocardium by technetium-99m-MIBI imaging after nitrate administration in chronic coronary artery disease. J Nucl Med 1995; 36: 1945–52.
9. Thorley PJ, Sheard KL, Wright DJ, Sivananthan UM. The routine use of sublingual GTN with resting 99Tcm-tetrofosmin myocardial perfusion imaging. Nucl Med Commun 1998; 19: 937–42.

6

Image processing

PRESENTATION OF MYOCARDIAL PERFUSION IMAGES

Single photon emission computed tomography (SPECT) slices should always be presented in a standard format for reporting. It is important always to use the same parameters, for example:

- number of slices
- magnification/zoom
- color scale
- degree of background subtraction.

Scans are reported by comparing a particular scan to a normal scan template – either the mental 'normal template' of the reporter or a normal database. This can only be achieved if the scans are always presented in the same format and one which the reporter is familiar with.

It is necessary to display short, vertical long axis, and horizontal long axis slices so that the whole of the left ventricle can be examined. The number of slices displayed depends on the particular software package used, but should always be the same once a protocol has been established. It is possible to customise some software but some packages do not allow this. Writing your own software to display slices is possible, but this must be fully documented, be rigorously tested, and comply with TickIT standards (http://www.tickit.org/) if this involves more than putting together commercially supplied commands.

Convention is to present images as shown in Figure 6.1, with stress slices as the top row, rest slices as the bottom row, for each set of slices. Short axis slices are from apex to base (left to right; L to R), vertical long axis slices from septum to lateral wall (L to R), and horizontal long axis slices from inferior to anterior (L to R). The anterior, inferior septal and lateral walls are as labelled. The format displayed here is that used on a Bartec system – other computer systems will have slightly different display formats. Images can also be displayed using a commercially available package which is independent of the camera/computer system. The slice display produced by one of the most commonly used packages, Cedars-Sinai Quantitative Perfusion SPECT (QPS),[1] is shown in Figure 6.2. Other frequently used packages are Emory Cardiac Toolbox[2] and 4D-MSPECT.[3]

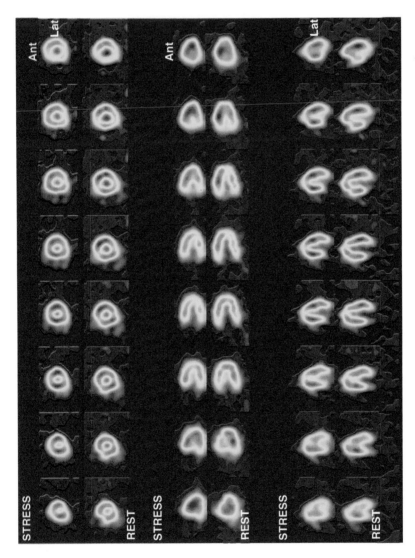

Figure 6.1 Normal scan showing the standard format for presentation of perfusion images. Short axis slices (top two rows) from apex to base reading from left to right, stress on top and rest underneath. The second two rows are the vertical long axis slices from septum to lateral wall, and the lower two rows are the horizontal long axis slices from inferior to anterior.

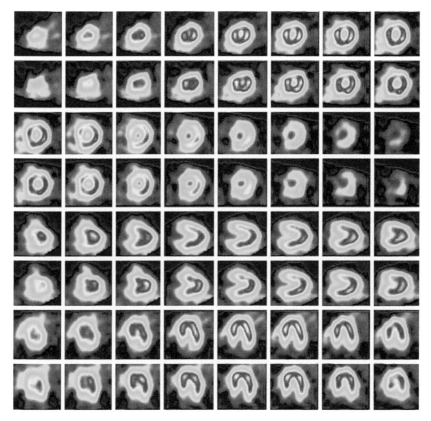

Figure 6.2 Normal myocardial perfusion scan presented using quantitative perfusion SPECT (QPS).

REVIEWING THE RAW DATA

During processing, it is important to look for and note any problems with the raw acquired data which may cause artefacts on the slice data. Although the images will have been reviewed after acquisition, it is not always possible to completely eliminate all problems, even with repeat imaging. A patient may still move even on a repeat scan, and they may, for example, have very large breasts, causing attenuation arte-facts. It is important to recognise the presence of attenuation and other artefacts at the processing stage so that they can be brought to the attention of the person report-ing the scan.

Movement

Artefacts due to movement will not usually be seen on the reconstructed slices if there is movement of less than 2 pixels on the raw data (for a 64-matrix acquisition).

The severity of the artefact will depend on the direction of the motion and whether it occurs once or many times throughout the acquisition. A very common motion artefact is seen on dual-headed cameras between the central projections when acquisition changes from one head to the other. This is due to gradual patient motion which is not easily picked up, but which is noticeable as a change in position between the beginning and end of the study (the last frame of one head and the first frame of the other head). Motion in the y direction (side to side or twisting motion) often causes a bigger artefact than motion in the x direction (head to foot motion). Figure 6.3 shows an artefact typical of this type of motion on the rest study, contrasted with the artefact-free stress study. The small anterior septal defect which is more apparent towards the apex can be attributed to patient movement.

Apical artefacts

It can be difficult to correctly position patients at acquisition if they are very large and/or have very dilated ventricles. The apex can be missed out of the acquisition field of view and a repeat scan should be performed. On reviewing the raw data it is important to check that an apical defect is not due to the apex being 'cut off' the acquired data. In some cases it may appear that the apex has just been included in the acquired images, but if the apex is very close to the edge of the field of view an artefact may be seen in the reconstructed slices, as shown in Figure 6.4. Here the apex appears to have more counts than the adjacent myocardium and has a very pointed appearance.

Gating errors – flash

When gating is performed, the patient's heart rate should be steady to ensure good data acquisition and to avoid artefacts in the summed data used to reconstruct the perfusion slices. Artefacts can occur if the heart rate fluctuates and beats are rejected. The introduction of artefacts is a possibility if 'flash' is seen when the summed data are viewed in cine mode. This is due to a change in image intensity between frames when beats have been rejected, leading to reduced counts if a fixed time per frame is used or a longer time per frame if a fixed number of beats per frame is used. This may either produce artefactual defects in the processed slices, or result in the obliteration of genuine defects. When this occurs, the acquisition should be repeated without gating.

Attenuation

A reduction in counts due to breast attenuation may be seen on the raw data, and it is important to look for reduced count density around the left ventricle due to breast tissue, as this may cause attenuation artefacts on the reconstructed slices. Figure 6.5 shows breast shadowing on the raw data. Attenuation defects are generally anterior, but if the breasts are very large, defects in other regions may also be seen.

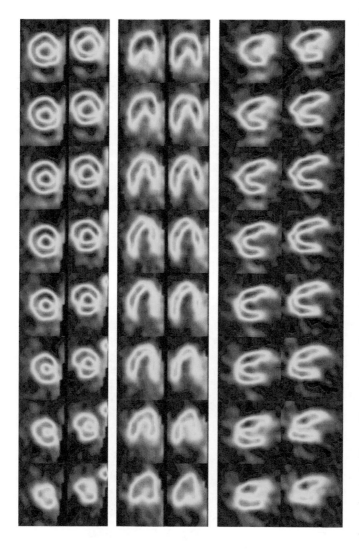

Figure 6.3 Stress and rest short axis slices with a motion artefact typical of gradual patient movement between the start and end of the study on the rest acquisition, with no motion during the stress study. The small anterior septal defect which is more apparent towards the apex can be attributed to patient movement.

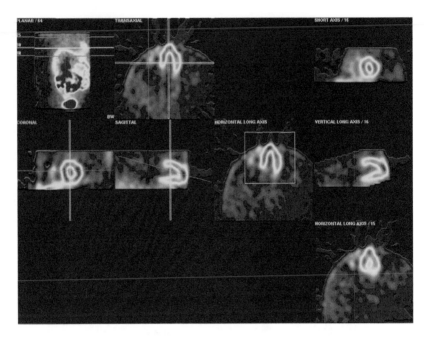

Figure 6.4 The left ventricle is positioned right at the edge of the field of view (first image) and in the reconstructed slices the apex appears to have more counts than the adjacent myocardium and has a very pointed appearance.

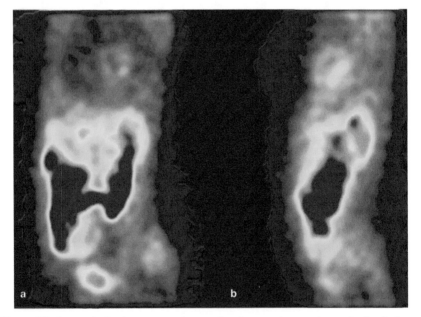

Figure 6.5 Breast shadowing seen on the raw data images. An anterior projection is shown in (a) with a large area of low counts above and to both sides of the left ventricle due to over-lying breast tissue. The extent of the breast is shown in the lateral view (b).

PROCESSING THE RAW DATA

This section will go through the necessary stages for manual processing of the raw data. Automatic processing packages will be discussed later. It is important to know what is happening at each stage, even if this is done automatically.

Production of slices

There are two ways of producing the axial slices from the acquired data – filtered back-projection (FBP) and iterative reconstruction. Historically, FBP was the method most widely used, as iterative reconstruction took too much computing time for routine use. However, mathematical techniques have been vastly improved, and iterative reconstruction is now widely available and quick to use.

FBP is a mathematical technique used to create images from a set of multiple projection profiles. It essentially involves 'correcting' the projection profiles by convolving them with a suitable mathematical filter and then back-projecting the filtered projections into image space. Camera computer systems usually have empirically determined optimal filters set up by the manufacturer for the particular SPECT myocardial perfusion protocol used. Different filters may be used for different acquisition matrix sizes, and different filters may be used for gated data compared to perfusion data. It is possible to change these for user-defined filters, but these should again be empirically designed to give the particular smoothing and detail required.

Filters used in FBP of myocardial perfusion images

Filters are described by a filter name – for example Butterworth, Hanning, Metz – and a critical (cut-off) frequency. Butterworth and Hanning filters (which are the ones most commonly used in myocardial perfusion scintigraphy) are low pass filters. This means that low frequencies (corresponding to large uniform objects) are allowed in the filtered image but high frequencies are reduced. High frequencies correspond to small objects or edges and noise. The effect of low pass filtering is to smooth the data and reduce noise, but there will also be a loss of edge definition and small detail. Decreasing the filter cut-off will cause very smooth images with loss of detail and contrast resolution, and will decrease the sensitivity for detection of perfusion abnormalities. On the other hand, increasing the cut-off value will accentuate high frequency data and exaggerate noise. This will reduce image quality, making it difficult to decide what constitutes a true defect and making those defects appear larger. For a 64 by 64 matrix acquisition and 64 angles, a commonly used filter is a Butterworth of order 5 and cut-off of 0.25 cycles/pixel. Cut-off values can also be expressed as cycles/cm or as a fraction of the Nyquist frequency (which is 0.5 cycles/pixel), so it is important to check which units are used when comparing filters.

Metz filters can also be used for myocardial perfusion imaging. A Metz filter is an adaptive or restoration filter, rather than a low pass filter. This means that the filter can

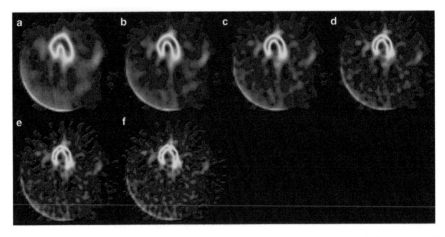

Figure 6.6 A single filtered back-projection (FBP) slice produced using different cut-off values for the Butterworth filter. As the cut-off increases (from a to f) the images become less smooth, but some fine detail may be lost at low cut-off values.

both amplify and attenuate different ranges of frequencies as selected by the user, and potentially can both reduce noise and maintain resolution. However, in practice the Metz filter is not as frequently used as the Butterworth as it is has a tendency to introduce artefacts into the image, and there is little difference in clinical image quality at the low count densities seen in myocardial perfusion imaging. Figure 6.6 shows a single FBP slice produced using a Butterworth filter, using different cut-off values. As the cut-off decreases, the images become smoother, but some fine detail is lost.

In gated SPECT the choice of filter is particularly important, as the calculated ejection fraction (EF) and ventricular volume values will depend to some extent on the filter used. As the gated data have a lower count density compared to the summed data used to obtain the perfusion slices, the best results may be obtained if a slightly less sharp filter is used to reconstruct the gated slices. A filter which has a cut-off value of 0.05 less than that used for the perfusion data is recommended.

Data should be filtered before back-projection. Theoretically, this is more effective than filtering during back-projection, as noise is reduced at the start of image processing. It is important always to use the same filter for a particular set of acquisition parameters so that the reconstruction process will not influence image interpretation. For a 2-day scan the same dose is generally used, and the same acquisition parameters. For a 1-day scan protocol, different doses are used at stress and rest, and so the counts/pixel are different. However, the same filter is normally used for both.

Iterative reconstruction

Iterative reconstruction is an algebraic technique which uses the projection data to produce an exact mathematical solution to the activity distribution from which the projection data come. The value of each pixel in the reconstruction is treated as an

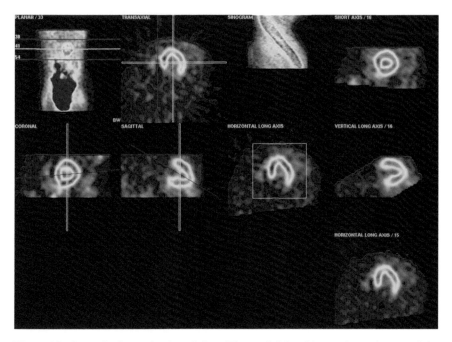

Figure 6.7   Stages in the production of slices. The top left hand image shows the area of the image which is reconstructed (between the red lines) and the reconstructed slice level (green line). The other images show the re-orientation angles used for producing short and long axis slices from the transaxial slices and the reconstructed slices. Also shown is the sinogram for the particular slice used.

unknown value, and each point in a profile as an equation. An initial estimate of the pixel values is made (usually, but not always, using filtered back-projection), and the initial values are altered slightly several times (iterations) until a final result is produced which is consistent with the count profiles. The number of iterations varies as does the precise mathematical technique used, but commonly used software employs between 4 and 10 iterations and OSEM (ordered subsets expectation maximization). The advantage of iterative reconstruction is that it can take account of attenuation and scatter if these are known, so when attenuation correction is used, reconstruction should always be performed using iterative techniques. There are also suggestions that even without attenuation correction, image quality is superior when iterative reconstruction rather than FBP is used.

Filtering, orientation and scaling of slices

Because the heart lies obliquely within the chest, reorientation is necessary to produce true short and long axis slices through the left ventricle. Regardless of the software used, and whether manual or automatic processing systems are employed, the same basic steps are involved. These are listed below and shown in Figure 6.7:

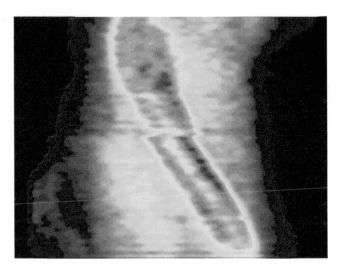

Figure 6.8   Sinogram showing significant patient movement with a discontinuity in the sinogram at the point where data from head 1 changes to data from head 2 for an acquisition with a dual-headed camera.

1. Set upper and lower limits either side of the myocardium before filtering. Adjust the saturation level until the myocardium is clearly seen.
2. Filter the data.
3. Set the slice to be reconstructed to the centre of the left ventricle (green line on Figure 6.7).
4. Check for movement by producing the sinogram for the chosen slice. A sinogram is a two-dimensional image of the projection data for a single slice for all the projection angles, in this case for the slice at the centre of the left ventricle (green line). If there is significant patient movement one or more discontinuities will be seen in the sinogram. Figure 6.8 shows a sinogram with significant patient movement between frames 32 and 33 (from head 1 to head 2 on a dual-headed camera).
5. Zoom if required. If data are acquired on a 128 matrix, it can be zoomed at this stage to a 64 by 64 matrix. Zooming may also be necessary if the left ventricle is very small.
6. Back-project to produce a transaxial slice.
7. Re-orient the slice to the vertical position with the apex at the top of the image in Figure 6.7.
8. Re-orient the slices in the coronal and sagittal planes to produce short and long axis slices. Re-orientation of the coronal view is difficult, as the only landmark is to try and set the reconstruction plane at right angles to the right ventricle. Usually this is close to the horizontal. It is important not to use too big an angle of correction as artefacts can be produced, as shown in Figure 6.9.

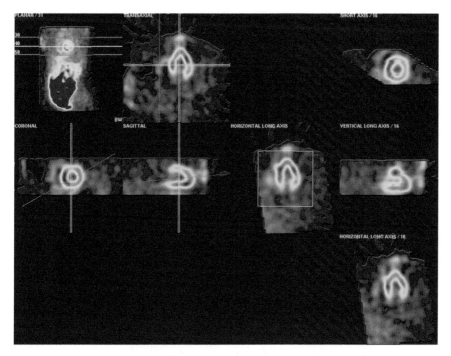

Figure 6.9   Slice production as in Figure 6.7 but with the coronal reconstruction plane set at too large an angle. Artefacts are seen as a horizontal line pattern on the reconstructed slices.

9. Check through the short horizontal long axis and vertical long axis slices and save (and label) these as sets of stress or rest slices if correct. Process the rest slices first (may be higher uptake in ischaemia) then the gated slices if done at rest, and then the stress slices using the same axes for orientation. However, if patient positioning was not exactly the same at stress and rest, slight adjustment of the axes may be required.

10. Align the stress and rest images so that the equivalent myocardial slices are paired at stress and rest. The processing system shown in Figure 6.1 allows eight short axis, horizontal long axis and vertical long axis images to be displayed at both stress and rest. This displays most of the left ventricle (except the very apical and very basal short axis slices) in a patient with a normal sized one. It is not always possible to align the images exactly due to the limited number of slices produced. Figure 6.10 shows the same stress and rest short axis slices with slightly different alignment. The rest short axis slices in the bottom set are aligned one slice further to the right than in the top set of slices. Neither choice of alignment is perfect and an intermediate solution is not possible.

    Large ventricles. In some patients the left ventricle is so large that a better representation of the whole of the left ventricle on the eight display frames is obtained by displaying every other slice rather than contiguous slices. This is shown in Figure 6.11.

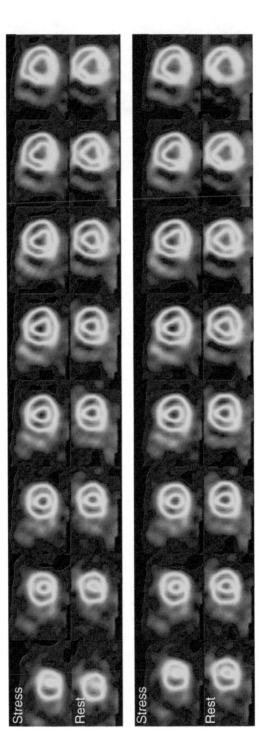

Figure 6.10 Short axis slices which are slightly misaligned. The rest short axis slices in the bottom pair of images are aligned one slice further to the right than in the top pair of images, compared to the same stress slices. Neither choice is perfect as the best alignment would require an intermediate solution, which is not possible.

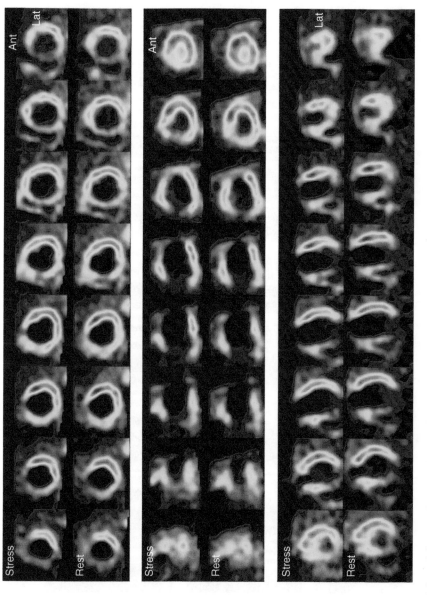

Figure 6.11 A large left ventricle (LV) is displayed as alternate slices rather than contiguous slices.

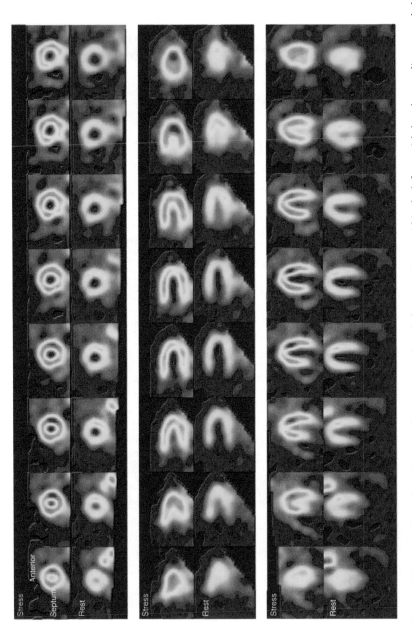

Figure 6.12 Short and long axis slices where the stress slices are correctly scaled to a maximum within the left ventricle but the rest slices are scaled to a maximum in the bowel.

11. Set the maximum scale value. The stress and rest slices should be scaled separately to the maximum count in the left ventricle in the stress and rest data set respectively. This is usually done automatically during computer processing of the slices. Counts in the left ventricle should be similar at stress and rest for a 2-day protocol using the same dose, but will differ when different doses are used as in a 1-day protocol. If the maximum count lies outside the left ventricle (due to liver/bowel uptake, for example), the scaling may need to be manually adjusted so that the perfusion does not appear globally reduced in the left ventricle on the set of slices where this is a problem. This is illustrated in Figure 6.12, where the stress slices are correctly scaled to a maximum within the left ventricle but the rest slices are scaled to a maximum in the bowel. The rest slices need re-scaling to enable a correct comparison between stress and rest. Figure 6.13 shows the same data as Figure 6.12 but with the rest slices scaled to the left ventricle.

Bowel/liver very close/overlying the left ventricle

If bowel/liver overlies the inferior wall of the left ventricle producing a 'hot' area, this may mean that the rest of the left ventricular uptake appears reduced. The scaling may need to be adjusted so that the inferior wall is oversaturated, but as the inferior wall has overlying extracardiac activity this area is non-diagnostic in any case. This is shown in Figure 6.14. Very high uptake just below the left ventricle may also cause a problem due to a reconstruction artefact when using filtered back-projection. High extracardiac activity may result in apparently reduced uptake adjacent to this in the inferior wall of the left ventricle. This is not a problem with iterative reconstruction.

Hot spots

Uptake in the left ventricle is sometimes very inhomogeneous. There may appear to be a 'hot spot' in the left ventricle. Manual rescaling to oversaturate the hot spot may then be required. This should be done cautiously, as it may not be a 'hot spot' but globally reduced perfusion elsewhere in the ventricle, and two sets of image data – scaled to maximum count and rescaled – should be presented for reporting. This is shown in Figure 6.15 where there appears to be a 'hot spot' in the septum at stress.

Choice of colour table

A colour scheme which is continuous, with a linear change between colours, should be used. An example of such a colour scale is the popular red, green and blue one used in the figures for this chapter. The colour scale should allow defects to be easily perceived, but without showing too much noise. Greyscale images are not used in myocardial perfusion studies, as defects are more easily seen using an appropriate colour table.

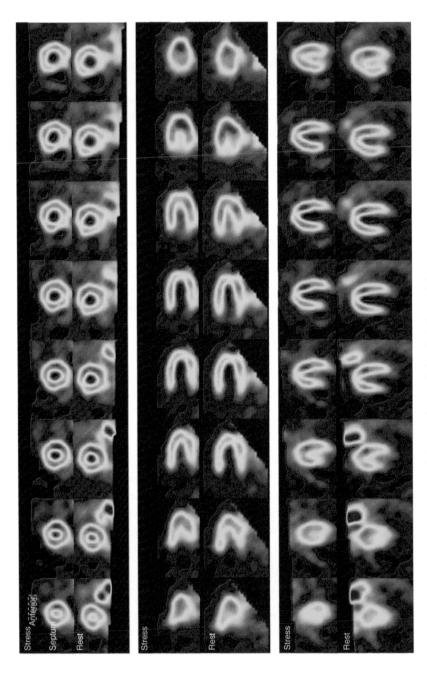

Figure 6.13 The same data as Figure 6.12 but with the rest slices scaled to the left ventricle.

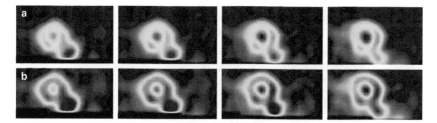

Figure 6.14   Short axis slices with bowel overlying the inferolateral region at stress. The slices in (a) are scaled to bowel while those in (b) are scaled to oversaturate the bowel and the infero-lateral region of the left ventricle but making the rest of the left ventricle more visible.

Background subtraction

When preparing images for reporting, background subtraction should not be used. Images should be presented in the same way for all patients, and this is far easier to achieve when background subtraction is avoided. High background levels can also be an indication of low myocardial uptake, which is useful information for the person reporting the scan.

Automatic processing packages

Automatic processing packages are available on a number of camera/computer systems. These will automatically set the angles required to produce short and long axis slices during the reconstruction process. These packages work well on normal data but may fail when there are large perfusion defects, so it is very important to check the resulting slices and manually adjust the angles if required. It may also be necessary to alter the angles between the stress and rest studies if patient positioning was slightly different on the two acquisitions, as the spatial orientation of the axes will be different.

SEMIQUANTITATIVE ANALYSIS

Polar plots

Polar plots are parametric images (where pixel values are related to the value of a parameter – in this case maximum count profiles rather than count density) which can be produced from the short axis slices only or the whole data set, depending on the software used. Polar plots give a single image which shows the whole data set at stress or rest and can be a useful overview. They can also be used for further analysis – either a form of segmental analysis as shown in Figure 6.16 or for comparison to a normal database of polar plots.

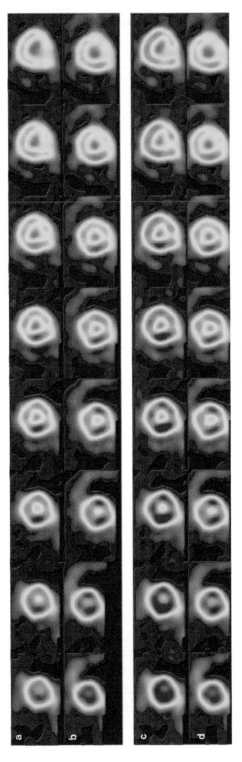

Figure 6.15   Short axis slices with a 'hot spot' in the septum at stress. Slices (a) and (c) are the same stress slices and (b) and (d) the same rest slices. The stress slices in (a) appear to show reduced counts towards the base of the left ventricle, while slices in (c) are re-scaled to oversaturate the septum, but the basal slices now appear similar in counts to the basal rest slices.

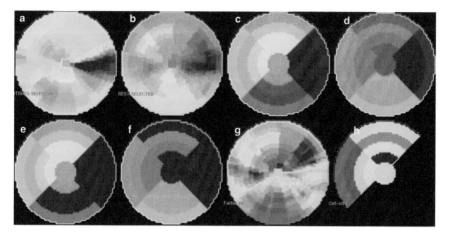

Figure 6.16   Polar plots at stress (a) and rest (b), and 17-segment analysis for the stress (c) and rest images (d). Imposition of normal cut-off values is shown in (e) and (f) for stress and rest, with red segments being in the normal range. Images (g) and (h) show a significant increase in perfusion at rest compared to stress in the anterior and septal regions.

Production of polar plots

The apex and base of the left ventricle are defined either manually or automatically, and the left ventricle between these boundaries is used to produce the polar plots. Radii (typically 60 at 6° intervals) are constructed from the centre to the base and are used to generate maximum-count profiles from the apex to the base which are mapped into successive rings in the polar map (the apex is mapped into the centre and the base is mapped into the periphery). Each ring within the polar map is assigned the same width in pixels. It is important to set the apex and base quite accurately, and in particular not to include too much base, especially with small ventricles, as erroneous basal defects may then be produced.

Segmental analysis

The left ventricle is divided into a number of segments (17 in Figure 6.16), and the segment with the maximum counts per pixel at stress is set at 100% and the other segments in the stress polar plot are calculated as percentages of this maximum. In the rest polar plot, the segments are scaled to the same segment which was used in the stress plot, even if it is not the hottest at rest. Further analysis is possible with the imposition of normal cut-off values (70% of maximum, for example), and any segments below normal can be displayed. Segments which 'improve' at rest can also be displayed, as an indication of regions of possible reversible ischaemia. It can be very useful to look at the polar plots and see whether these apparently reversible defects can be confirmed by examination of the slice data.

Comparison to a normal database

Polar plots can also be compared to an idealised normal polar plot, and any areas which show reduced uptake can be identified. It is possible to produce a normal polar plot from data acquired on your own camera/computer system, but more common to use a commercially available myocardial perfusion quantitative package. Separate normal polar plots are required for males and females because of the effects of attenuation. If attenuation correction is used, then a single normal polar plot can be used.

MYOCARDIAL PERFUSION QUANTITATIVE PACKAGES

Software packages are used to quantify myocardial perfusion images as they can improve accuracy and reduce inter- and intraobserver variation in reporting. They are particularly useful for inexperienced reporters. Quantitation is not absolute – it is not possible at present with SPECT to quantify myocardial perfusion in terms of absolute blood flow, or to measure accurately the effects of attenuation and scatter. These software packages compare data to normal templates (after scaling) and show the location of a defect, and whether or not it improves at rest, and may indicate the extent and severity of a defect.

There are three main packages currently available:

- Cedars-Sinai Quantitative Perfusion SPECT (QPS)
- Emory Cardiac Toolbox (ECTb)
- 4D-MSPECT.

To enable these package to work, data must be of reasonable quality; in particular there must be no high activity extracardiac uptake close to the myocardium. If there is high activity in the liver or bowel close to or overlapping the myocardium, then manual identification of the myocardial edges will be required, and results may be inaccurate. The packages require the input of reconstructed short and long axis slices at stress and rest. Stress and rest slices are then automatically aligned, with the option to manually adjust if required. Polar plots are calculated from the aligned slices and comparison made to a normal database using a 17- or 20-segment model and a 5-point scoring system, where 0 = normal uptake, 1 = mildly reduced, 2 = moderately reduced, 3 = severely reduced, and 4 = absent. Each segment is separately scored, and then a summed stress score, summed rest score and summed difference score can be obtained. Patients can then be classified on the basis of these scores as normal (score < 4), mildly abnormal (4–8), moderately abnormal (9–13), and severely abnormal (> 13). Normal databases are sex-specific and isotope-specific, and there may be separate databases for 1- and 2-day technetium protocols. The appearance of a 'normal' scan will depend to some extent on the camera/computer system used and the acquisition and processing protocols. The most accurate results will be obtained using a local normal database. It has been possible to generate user-specific normal databases using QPS, but this requires large numbers of normal and abnormal scans with defects in specific segments, and so is difficult to set up. The latest version of QPS has a simpler method of establishing your own normal database, which should be more useful, and may improve the accuracy of the quantitation.

Defect extent and severity

The software packages will calculate the extent of a defect and its severity, which may help to decide whether it is clinically significant, and can be useful in assigning prognostic significance to perfusion abnormalities.

It is important to note that although all packages quantify perfusion abnormalities, they will each give different results. It is therefore only possible to compare results of different examinations on the same patient if the same processing software was used on each occasion. When reporting, quantitative results are used in conjunction with a visual interpretation of the slice data (see Chapter 7).

PROCESSING OF GATED SLICES

Gated data may be acquired at rest, at stress or for both acquisitions. In either case, the patient is likely to be in a resting state by the time the data are acquired, even if the injection was actually administered at peak stress, and so any functional parameters derived from them will reflect the position at rest. Gated data are first summed and the stress or rest slices produced in the usual way. Gated slices then need to be produced, and this is best done immediately after the perfusion images have been derived, using the same angulation for the reconstructions. Once gated slices have been produced they can be simply viewed to look at wall motion and thickening, but a commercial package should be used to obtain quantitative values of ejection fraction (EF) and left ventricular volumes. Currently available packages include:

- Cedars-Sinai Quantitative Gated SPECT (QGS)[4]
- Emory Cardiac Toolbox (ECTb)[5]
- 4D-MSPECT.[6]

These packages are very simple to use and automatically calculate EF and left ventricular volumes from the gated data. The automatic processing will fail if there is high intensity extracardiac activity (liver or bowel) very close to the inferior wall of the ventricle, as shown in Figure 6.17. In such cases it may be possible to define the left ventricle outline manually to obtain quantitative functional information. In order to obtain accurate values for EF and ventricular volumes it is important that there are reasonable levels of activity in the myocardium. Where this is not the case,

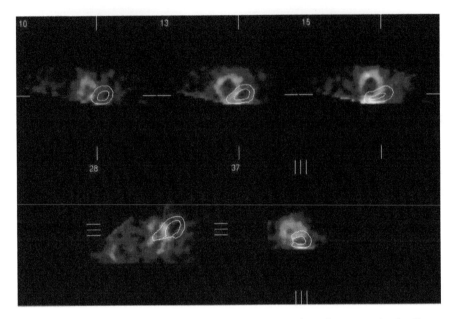

Figure 6.17 Quantitative gated SPECT (QGS) processing where the automatic edge detection has failed due to high bowel activity adjacent to the inferior wall of the left ventricle. Note that the thermal colour scale is used.

for example in studies where there is high attenuation, extensive ischaemia, or a generalised abnormality such as cardiomyopathy, the software may have difficulty detecting the edges of the ventricle, and quantitative results will be subject to more error than usual. Comparisons of EF measurements obtained using gated SPECT data with those from other imaging techniques and modalities such as radionuclide ventriculography and magnetic resonance imaging (MRI) show them to be accurate and reproducible. However, similar comparisons of estimates of ventricular volume show poorer correlation, and the SPECT values may not be sufficiently accurate and reproducible for repeat studies. It is important, as with all such techniques, to establish a normal range for the particular camera, computer, and acquisition and processing protocols used. Different normal ranges for volumes may be required for women as they have smaller hearts. Normal ranges for EF are not dependent on sex.

Small hearts

Gated SPECT processing packages will give erroneously high EFs and low volumes in patients with small hearts with end-diastolic volume (EDV) less than about 70 ml. These patients are usually female, and this is due to difficulty in accurately detecting the edges of such small ventricles. Problems are reduced if the pixel size at acquisition is about 5 mm, which may require zooming.

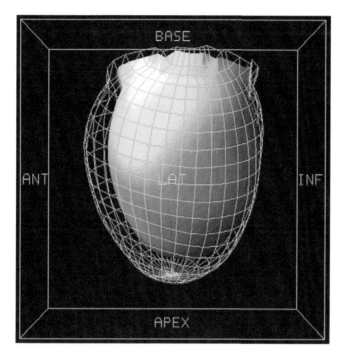

Figure 6.18 QGS image demonstrating normal anterior wall motion but an akinetic inferior wall. The green mesh is end diastole and the blue shading indicates the inner wall of the left ventricle at systole.

Wall motion and wall thickening

Slice data can be displayed in cine mode to assess wall thickening using a colour display, and wall motion using a linear grey scale. It is possible to view the three-dimensional images produced by the software in cine mode to look at the ventricle from any angle, and so get an overall idea of wall motion. Figure 6.18 shows a still image from such a display, with a normal anterior wall but akinetic inferior wall. The software packages will also score wall motion and thickening against a normal database. QGS, for example, assigns movement scores of 0=normal, 1=mild hypokinesia, 2=moderate hypokinesia, 3=severe hypokinesia, 4=akinesia, and 5=dyskinesia, and wall thickening is scored from 0 (normal) to 3 (severely reduced). Some software will also give values for wall motion and wall thickening in mm and %, which is useful for repeat studies to see whether there has been improvement following treatment. It is important to know what constitutes a significant change, and what is normal for different ventricular regions. The septum usually appears to move less well compared to the free wall, and there may be some apparent reduction in wall motion right at the base of the heart. Thus, normal wall motion and wall thickening are not uniform across the ventricle.

REFERENCES

1. Germano G, Kavanagh PB, Waechter P et al. A new algorithm for the quantitation of myocardial perfusion SPECT. I: technical principles and reproducibility. J Nucl Med 2000; 41: 712–19.
2. Van Train KF, Areeda J, Garcia EV et al. Quantitative same-day rest-stress technetium-99m-sestamibi SPECT: definition and validation of stress normal limits and criteria for abnormality. J Nucl Med 1993; 34: 1494–502.
3. Ficaro EP, Kritsman JN, Corbett JR. Development and clinical validation of normal Tc-99m sestamibi database: comparison of 3D-MSPECT to Cequal. J Nucl Med 1999; 40: 125.
4. Germano G, Kiat H, Kavanagh PB et al. Automatic quantification of ejection fraction from gated myocardial perfusion SPECT. J Nucl Med 1995; 36: 2138–47.
5. Faber TL, Cooke CD, Folks RD et al. Left ventricular function and perfusion from gated perfusion images: an integrated method. J Nucl Med 1999; 40: 650–9.
6. Chugh A, Ficaro EP, Moscucci M et al. Quantification of left ventricular function by gated perfusion tomography: testing of a new fully automatic algorithm. J Am Coll Cardiol 2001; 37: 394A.

7
Myocardial perfusion scintigraphy: interpretation and reporting

GENERAL ISSUES

The preceding chapters have introduced the key concepts underpinning the use of myocardial perfusion scintigraphy (MPS), and explained how to set up and run a nuclear cardiology service. This chapter assumes that everything has gone well, and that you are now producing high-quality images of the myocardium at stress and rest, hopefully with electrocardiogram (ECG) gating. Although we have to interpret the images before producing a report (hence the title of this chapter), we will reverse that order and begin by addressing a number of important general issues around reporting before launching into a systematic discussion of image interpretation.

Who does the reporting?

When this 'who does what' type of question is raised in the healthcare setting, the answer, increasingly frequently, is that it does not matter as long as they have the proper training. The days when particular tasks were jealously guarded by one professional group or another are fast receding, and activities that used to be the sole preserve of doctors are being taken on by non-medically qualified health professionals under the guise of 'role extension' or 'skills mix'. Radionuclide imaging reporting is performed variously by nuclear medicine physicians, radiologists, medical physicists, nuclear medicine technicians and radiographers and, in the case of MPS, by cardiologists. What is important is that reporters are adequately trained. In the case of MPS, that has to include a significant amount of clinical training and experience in order to have the necessary understanding of the background to the referral and the possible implications of the report for the patient. That does not necessarily mean that only medically qualified people can report myocardial perfusion studies; I know at least one radiographer who has worked so long in nuclear cardiology, liaising closely with cardiologists, that she is as well able to report a scan as I am. However, it is likely that most reporting will be performed by clinicians (and I do of course include radiologists in that definition!).

In all areas of diagnostic radiology or nuclear medicine, close cooperation with referring clinicians is important, and that is clearly the case for MPS. It is possible to report MPS examinations in isolation, never meeting a cardiologist or obtaining feedback on the patients whose scans you have reported. However, this is professionally unsatisfying, and is unlikely to result in an optimal service to either the patient or the referring clinician. It is even more important to have contact with cardiologists during the training phase. It is only by discussing patients with them, and seeing how the MPS report influences management, that you can develop a reporting style that meets their cardiological needs. It is also the case that the best way to learn where to set diagnostic thresholds and avoid over- or under-reporting (see below) is by seeing reports utilised in a clinical setting and weighed alongside the results of other investigations. Dual reporting by imaging specialist and cardiologist might be a counsel of perfection which is seldom attainable, but regular joint review of difficult patients either on an occasional basis or at a regular meeting is a very good second best.

Hard copy or soft copy?

The type of display used is an important variable in reporting. Most of us now sit in front of a workstation to view images, rather than looking at hard copy. This represents an enormous advance in many ways, but it is a two-edged sword. When we only had hard copy to look at, we were at the mercy of the radiographer or technician who produced it, not to mention the performance of the hard copy device itself. Although it was possible to reprint images which were clearly technically inadequate, it involved considerable effort, and sometimes it was not even apparent that there had been a problem at the hardcopying stage. Now we can flick back and forth between sets of images, apply different processing algorithms at the touch of a button, and alter display parameters as much and as often as we like. However, it is important that each centre establishes its standard display criteria (particularly colour tables) at an early stage, and sticks with them while building up experience with a particular computer system and software. It is soon possible to get a feel for how much manipulation is acceptable and helpful, and when it begins to detract from the information content of the image. In this way it is possible to avoid what has been described as the 'dial a defect' syndrome.

Quantitative or qualitative?

As we will see below, MPS images do not just contain diagnostic information; they are subject to artefact – both patient-generated (attenuation; movement) and those arising from the acquisition and processing systems. When reporting, we have to differentiate artefact from pathology, and if we believe that we have detected a genuine abnormality, decide whether to report it at all and, if so, how much significance to attribute to it. The key factor in producing an accurate report is the combination of high quality images and an experienced eye. Quantitative information from polar plots and other automated assessment of the images (Chapter 6) can be useful in reducing the subjective element in interpretation and increasing the reporter's confidence in decision-making, but it is possible to place undue reliance on numerical data. Quantitative analyses of images are subject to errors resulting from artefact or statistical fluctuations in the input data which may not be immediately apparent when looking at the report screen, and the key element in arriving at a conclusion has to be experienced visual assessment of the images, weighted by full consideration of the clinical context and the results of other investigations (notably angiography). This approach is rather grandly designated as 'quantitative imaging with visual over-read', which tends to mean that you treat the quantitative data with respect, but ignore them when they conflict with clinical common sense.

One of the most important contributions of quantitative data is to improve the reproducibility of results and reduce inter- and intraobserver variation. This is particularly important in research and in the extraction of prognostic information from MPS data, where semiquantitative segmental scoring systems can be useful (see 'Image interpretation' below). The reason that quantitation is often of only limited assistance in coming to a diagnostic conclusion on individual studies is that the programs are using the same image data that you have been looking at. The patients we need most help with are those where the images are giving us an equivocal message. Feed that data into a computer program, and it is likely that the quantitative result of the processing will also fall into the grey area between normal and abnormal.

Is gating worthwhile?

The technique of gating has been described earlier, and the short answer to the question posed here is 'yes'. So it is worrying that, at the time of writing, fewer than a quarter of the MPS examinations carried out in the UK employ gating. Everything that follows in this chapter will assume that a technetium-labelled radiopharmaceutical is used, and that a gated acquisition has been performed (gated single photon emission computed tomography (SPECT) using the doses of thallium allowed in the UK is difficult but not impossible). Hopefully, the information provided in this chapter will still be useful to centres not performing gated imaging, but it will rapidly become apparent that a non-gated study is an incomplete study. Gated data enable the reporter to differentiate more easily between fixed defects due to attenuation and those due to infarction, and also play a key role in providing prognostic information by allowing assessment of left ventricular function. Regional wall motion is also an important factor when assessing viability (see below).

Key point   Gated acquisition

Adds time to the study, but is a key component of MPS
Advantages:

- Aids the identification of defects due to attenuation
- Gives prognostic information
- Is important in the assessment of viability

Using all the data

MPS studies generate a lot of data. At the time of reporting, you may be viewing the reconstructed perfusion images, the polar (bull's-eye) display, and a gated acquisition with assessment of myocardial contractility and thickening, along with the associated quantitative data. This represents much information and can take a considerable amount of time. However, it is also important to view the raw images from which all of these data are derived, and this should be the first step in the reporting process. There is an information technology aphorism which states: 'rubbish in; rubbish out'. In other words, if there are deficiencies in the input data to any computing operation, the output will also be flawed. Inspection of the initial projections will help to identify potential sources of error, notably patient movement and attenuation (see below). It will also demonstrate and localise subdiaphragmatic activity, and identify any increase in lung activity. Of course, if the same person is processing and reporting the data, this step will take place at the processing stage. Often, though, the reporter will be viewing preprocessed data, and it is vital that they are aware of any quality issues with the raw data, and any steps taken to improve matters. For further discussion of this topic, see Chapter 6.

Reporting style

Setting a threshold for abnormality

Radiologists and nuclear medicine physicians are well aware of the fact that although the envelope containing the scan results is addressed to the referring clinician, it is actually the patient who is on the receiving end of their reports. Nowhere is this more relevant than in the case of nuclear cardiology. In the comfort (or squalor) of the reporting room, cut off from the bustle of the hospital, it is easy to become preoccupied with the image in front of you, and the need to produce a report that wrings every bit of information from it. However, no matter how much processing and quantification we apply to image data (see above), there is a large subjective element involved in image interpretation, and reporting a cardiac scan is as much an art as it is a science. We all have different thresholds for both perceiving abnormalities and ascribing significance to them, and radiologists (and anyone else who reports images for a living) consequently exhibit natural variation in the degree to which they under- or over-report. This is not just an interesting observation on human nature, it has implications for the patient, implications which can be particularly acute in the case of myocardial perfusion scanning.

It is possible to make a conscious effort to vary your threshold for reporting an imaging investigation as abnormal, and this is sometimes necessary. When reporting images acquired as part of a screening programme, for example breast cancer screening using mammography, the expected incidence of the target abnormality is low, and it is important to maximise sensitivity at the expense of specificity in order to minimise the number of cancers that slip through the screening net. You will tend to over-report questionable abnormalities, secure in the knowledge that any false positives will be identified as such by further imaging and biopsy before the patient is subjected to any major intervention. When reporting a bone scan in a patient with newly diagnosed lung cancer, on the other hand, you will tend to under-report doubtful abnormalities, since an over-zealous and mistaken report of bone metastasis will deprive the patient of their only chance of curative treatment. The main aim of MPS is to determine whether or not the patient has ischaemic heart disease and to provide information on risk stratification, so the result of the scan is likely to play a key role in determining whether the patient is a candidate for fairly major intervention. The MPS report will need to differentiate between abnormality and artefact, and will also grade the severity of any defect thought to be genuine. This gives the reporter the opportunity to steer the referring clinician gently in one direction or another, and it is better to err on the side of under-reporting doubtful abnormalities. The dubious lesions will tend, by definition, to be at the milder end of the spectrum and of correspondingly low prognostic significance, and the patient is likely to be under continuing medical supervision in any case. An aggressive attitude to reporting will result in patients coming to angiography, angioplasty or even surgery unnecessarily. This is not only distressing and potentially hazardous for the patients concerned, but it will also bring the MPS technique into disrepute.

Key point Hitting the right note

Reporting every minor reduction in uptake as a defect will result in the over-investigation of normal patients, with loss of confidence in MPS and increased morbidity from unnecessary interventions

Minor defects which turn out to be genuine are likely to be of low prognostic significance, and 'missing' them is unlikely to affect the management of patients, or the clinical outcome

---

Avoiding indecision

The comment in the previous paragraph that 'it is probably better to err on the side of under-reporting doubtful abnormalities' should not, however, be used as a reason to hedge reports around with 'ifs' and 'maybes'. One of the worst faults in any author of imaging reports is to take up a position on the diagnostic fence. Most clinicians much prefer a radiologist or nuclear medicine physician who issues reports that reach a conclusion, accepting that they will sometimes be wrong, to one who habitually qualifies his or her reports without committing themselves to a diagnosis. There will of course be some occasions where it is necessary to issue an equivocal report, and in that case it is vital to be open about the problems, making the limitations of the study clear. Wherever possible, though, reach a definite decision regarding the presence or absence of an abnormality and its prognostic significance. For example, if there is a fixed inferior wall defect in a male patient with no history of infarction, and gated imaging shows normal wall movement and thickening in the area of the defect, simply report that the changes are due to attenuation and that there are no significant perfusion defects present. In fact, you only need to mention the defect at all, because the referring clinician will probably have access to a set of images, and may otherwise wonder if you had failed to see it. The combination of an indecisive report and a cautious clinician will result in an unacceptably high incidence of normal angiograms, and this will eventually lead to a loss of confidence in MPS as a technique, and in you as a colleague.

Structured report or free text?

This again is a matter of the personal style of the reporter, but I would make a plea for structured reporting. MPS reports tend to contain a lot of information, and presenting it simply as a block, or blocks, of uninterrupted text can result in some elements being missed by the clinician receiving the report. Breaking the report up into headed sections (for example: indications; stress protocol; perfusion images; gated study; and conclusion) makes it much more digestible. There is, of course, the risk that some clinicians will skip straight to the 'conclusion' section, but at least then they will have read the important part of the message.

Attributing defects to named vessels

Opinions differ on whether to report a defect simply in relation to the area of myocardium involved, or whether to attribute it to a specific vessel. Naming the vessel would be fine if coronary arterial anatomy was consistent, but as we know, the relative dominance of right and left main coronary arteries, and the area of myocardium subtended by each, can be very variable. Most reporters therefore describe defects in relation to the wall of the ventricle involved rather than the vessel. However, if a patient's angiogram reveals a 70% stenosis of uncertain significance in the left anterior descending artery (LAD) but normal circumflex and right coronary arteries, and if the scan shows an inducible defect in the anterior wall and septum, it would be unreasonably reticent not to attribute it to the LAD.

IMAGE INTERPRETATION

This section does not set out to be an exhaustive guide to the reporting of MPS scans, but it will hopefully serve as a useful introduction. There is no subsitute for sitting alongside an experienced reporter, and learning the trade under supervision.

The normal perfusion scan

Image presentation: perfusion images

The heart lies obliquely in the chest, and the precise orientation varies between patients. Consequently, the use of the standard anatomical planes (transverse, coronal, and sagittal) for reconstruction of cardiac tomographic slices would produce images in planes of varying obliquity which would be difficult to interpret, or to relate to vascular territories. To avoid this problem, processing software identifies the long axis of the left ventricle, and reconstructs short axis (SA) views perpendicular to this, then going on to reconstruct orthogonal horizontal and vertical long axis views (HLA and VLA – see Chapter 6).

These are typically presented as the SA stress views paired with the corresponding sections from the rest scan, followed by the paired HLA and VLA images. The SA views show the anterior wall of the ventricle at the top, inferior at the bottom, lateral wall to the right, and septum to the left. The HLA views are presented with the apex at the top, lateral wall to the right, and septum to the left. The VLA cuts have the apex to the right, anterior wall at the top, and inferior at the bottom (Figure 7.1a and b). Vascular territories can be mapped on to these sections (Figure 7.1c), but care has to be taken in assigning abnormalities to lesions in individual vessels, due to the considerable range of normal variation in coronary blood supply (see previous section).

As the initial steps in processing the data are to construct the true short axis sections perpendicular to the long axis of the ventricle and then use them to derive the HLA and VLA sections, there is clearly no information in the long axis views that is not present on the SA images. However, the HLA and VLA sections are useful in checking the appearances of the apex and, to a lesser extent, the base of the ventricle, where partial volume effects can be a problem. In particular, care should be taken in interpreting apical short axis slices where there is no, or very little, ventricular cavity visible. Any defects on these slices are very likely to be due to partial volume effects, or to the fact that the true apex is off the axis of rotation of the camera. Apical abnormalities must be assessed on the long axis views, for example when differentiating between apical thinning (below) and true defects.

Image presentation: polar images

Usually referred to as a bull's-eye plot, this display presents the short axis sections as rings of increasing diameter, with the apex at the centre and the base of the heart at the periphery. This allows quick assessment of the number and area of any defects at stress and rest. Comparison with a database of normal images will highlight areas of reduced activity which meet a predefined criterion for significance, and subtraction images can be produced to illustrate the extent of reversibility. Figure 7.2 shows a normal polar plot alongside examples of fixed and reversible defects.

Recognizing normality

One of the most important skills to acquire in imaging is that of recognizing normality, and the distribution of activity within the normal ventricular wall is not homogeneous. There are a number of common and identifiable areas of reduced uptake (see below), and on short axis views, the lateral wall typically shows the highest level of activity (Figure 7.3). This lack of uniformity is the reason that software packages for quantitative assessment of MPS studies compare the images with a locally produced database of

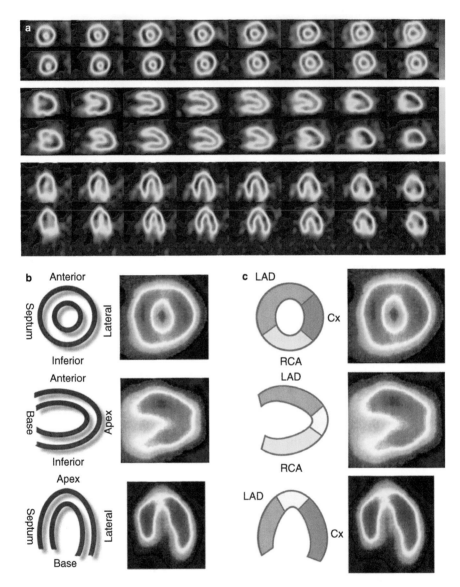

Figure 7.1 (a) Normal myocardial perfusion scintigraphy (MPS) study demonstrating the standard image display format. The top set of images are the short axis (SA) views, looking up the left ventricle from the apex, and the stress images are displayed above the corresponding sections from the rest study. The middle rows of images are the vertical long axis (VLA) views and at the bottom are the stress and rest horizontal long axis (HLA) views. Note that the septum is shorter than the lateral wall (see Figure 7.5). The right ventricle is barely visible on these window settings, a reflection of the much greater bulk of muscle in the thicker left ventricular wall. (b) SA, VLA and HLA views with diagrams identifying the walls of the ventricle visible on each projection. (c) Same projections, this time showing the vascular territories (LAD, left anterior descending; Cx, circumflex; RCA, right coronary artery). Potential cross-over territory at the apex is shown in yellow. But note that the areas subtended by these vessels are subject to significant anatomical variation (see text).

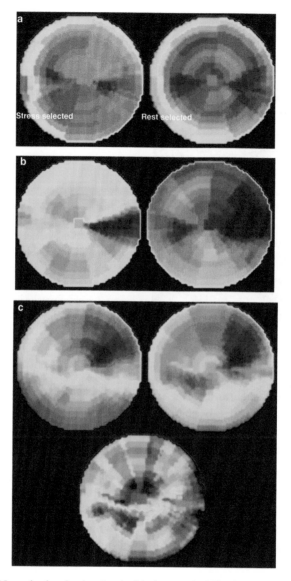

Figure 7.2 (a) Normal polar plot showing the SA views stacked like the rings in a tree trunk, with the apex at the centre and subsequent sections around this, extending out to the base of the ventricle at the periphery. (b) This plot shows a large reversible defect in the left anterior descending artery (LAD) territory. Note the extensive area of reduced uptake in the anterior wall and septum on the stress plot (left). Uptake in the inferior wall is also reduced when compared with the lateral wall. On the rest plot (right), there has been considerable recovery in the anterior wall and septum. (c) Polar plot showing a large fixed inferior defect with a smaller area of reversibility in the inferior part of the septum. Note the large inferior defect on the stress image (top left), the major part of which persists at rest (top right). The difference image (below) highlights the reversible component in the inferior septum, although this was easily appreciated by visual comparison of the stress and rest plots – an experienced eye is as good as most software programs in performing subtraction!

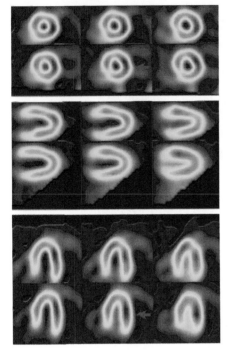

Figure 7.3 Views demonstrating the normal non-uniformity of uptake, with the lateral wall showing the highest level of activity (arrow), and the inferior wall the lowest. Levels of uptake in the normal inferior wall can be down to 80% of the maximum, and even less than that towards the base of the heart.

normal scans, highlighting areas where activity differs from normal by more than a pre-set threshold (for example, two standard deviations from the mean). The experienced observer does exactly the same, almost without thinking. There are three areas in particular which show a relative reduction in activity.

Inferior wall   The inferior wall is usually the coolest area. The range of variation does not normally exceed 20%, except towards the base of the heart, where it can approach 50%. This is enough to produce visible inhomogeneity, and it is important to recognise it as normal. The point at which this normal variation is designated as an attenuation defect (below) will vary from reporter to reporter.

Key point   Normal uptake is not homogeneous

It is important to develop an 'eye' for the normal variation of activity levels in the walls of the left ventricle:

- The lateral wall tends to be the hottest region
- The inferior wall is typically the coolest area, with levels of uptake around 80% of the maximum, or occasionally lower
- The septum appears shorter than the other walls, due to the absence of muscle in the membranous proximal portion
- Reduced apical uptake is often due to normal thinning and partial volume effects

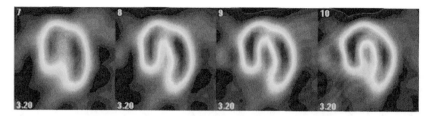

Figure 7.4 HLA view showing normal apical thinning. The decision that such a defect is normal is largely a matter of experience, and will depend on the clinical history; the size and severity of the defect; whether it is fixed or reversible; and the presence or absence of defects elsewhere. Apical defects should only be assessed on long axis views, as short axis images will be subject to partial volume effects in the apical region.

Apical thinning   It is also common to see a reduction in uptake at the apex, where the myocardium is thinner than elsewhere, and partial volume effects may also tend to minimise the amount of activity apparent (Figure 7.4). Again, it requires experience to get a feel for when this normal reduction becomes a genuine defect. The long axis views must be used when assessing apical abnormalities (see above).

Upper septum   The activity resides in the myocardium, and so it is normal to find a cold area in the membranous part of the interventricular septum, towards the base of the heart. This will result in absent septal activity in the basal short axis slices, but is best appreciated on the horizontal long axis views, where the shortness of the septum in relation to the lateral wall is clearly apparent (Figure 7.5).

Right ventricle   Because the right ventricular wall is thin in relation to that of the left ventricle, it is only faintly seen on a normal scan. Unusually prominent uptake in the right ventricle can be an important indicator of disease (see below).

Artefacts

Artefacts are a common feature of MPS images, and differentiating them from genuine defects is an important skill to acquire. The most frequent causes of artefact are attenuation and patient movement, but there are others.

Attenuation   Generally speaking, the bigger the patient, the more likely it is that attenuation will be a problem, but it can be seen in patients of any size. This is one reason to ensure that the height and weight of patients, and the bra size in women, are recorded, so that the person reporting the images can assess the likelihood that apparent abnormalities are due to attenuation. The anatomical structures most often responsible for attenuation artefacts are the diaphragm and the breast. By definition, attenuation defects should be fixed, and so the differential diagnosis is usually between attenuation and infarction. However, there can sometimes be some change

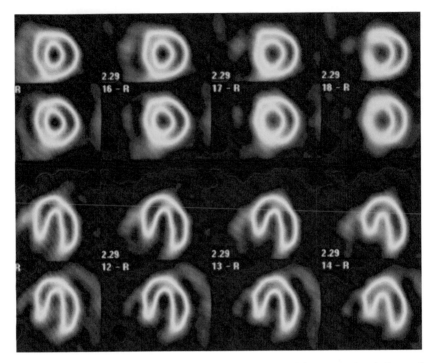

Figure 7.5   SA (top) and HLA views showing the shortness of the septum in relation to the lateral wall. This reflects the absence of muscle in the membranous upper portion of the septum. Clearly this should be a fixed defect, and it seldom if ever causes problems in interpretation of studies.

in appearance between stress and rest images even with attenuation, particularly when due to breast tissue (see below), which can make life really difficult. Attenuation correction software may be the answer in those patients where it proves difficult or impossible to decide whether a defect is genuine or artefactual, but it is not without its own problems (see below).

Diaphragmatic attenuation   This is a particular problem in male patients, but can occur in patients of either sex and any size. The defect produced is in the inferior wall, and represents an accentuation of the normal relative reduction in inferior counts described above (Figure 7.6). It is often fairly simple to recognise inferior wall attenuation for what it is by considering the patient's clinical history and the results of other investigations which may be available. For example, the patient may have had an angiogram which revealed a 60% stenosis of the left anterior descending artery but normal circumflex and right coronary arteries and a normal ECG, the only clinical question being the haemodynamic significance of the borderline LAD lesion. In that case it would be fairly safe to assume that a fixed inferior wall defect is due to attenuation rather than to infarction. However, life is not always that

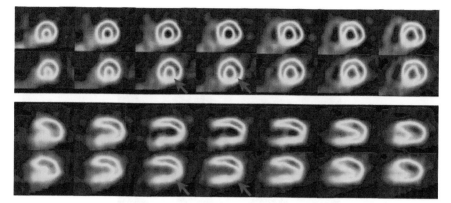

Figure 7.6 SA and VLA images showing inferior attenuation (arrows). This is really just a more extreme example of the 'normal' relative reduction in inferior uptake shown in Figure 7.3. As with apical thinning, the recognition that a defect is due to attenuation rather than a loss of perfusion is dependent on a number of factors, not least the size and weight of the patient; the clinical history and findings of other investigations; the absence of any other evidence of infarction or hibernation; and, critically, the results of gated imaging (see text).

simple, and it will often be difficult to decide from the images and clinical information alone whether such a defect is genuine or not. Changing the positioning of the patient may be helpful. Scanning with the patient prone instead of supine can reduce diaphragmatic attenuation, and we have had some success with this in the past. Some centres acquire additional left lateral planar views with the patient supine and then right side down, although we have no experience of this. We have found that the introduction of gated SPECT as a routine part of the scanning protocol is the most useful single measure for coping with attenuation artefacts. If there is a doubtful fixed defect which on gated imaging shows normal wall movement and thickening, we feel much safer in assuming it to be due to attenuation rather than infarction.

Breast attenuation   This is a common artefact in female patients (Figure 7.7). It should be recognised as a potential problem at the initial processing stage, where inspection of the raw images will reveal the shadow of the breast on the relevant projections (Figure 7.8). Here again, it tends to be in larger patients that breast attenuation is a particular problem, but it can be seen even in relatively slim women. Apparent reversibility can occur with breast attenuation, presumably due to the fact that the breasts are mobile. Some centres advise strapping them to reduce this effect, although even then it is difficult to ensure that the geometry is exactly the same on stress and rest images. We have tended to avoid strapping, and rely instead on reproducible positioning of the patient, in the hope that the unfettered breast will behave in a consistent fashion. Where the patient does wear a bra for the scan, we ask her to wear the same one for both visits. This time it is the anterior wall which is most affected, and as with diaphragmatic attenuation, the demonstration of normal

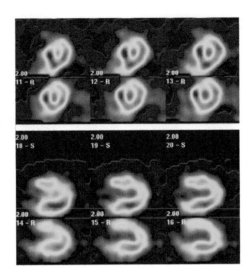

Figure 7.7   SA and VLA images showing breast attenuation. The reduction in uptake in the anterior wall is quite marked, and would be highly significant if due to ischaemia or infarction. However, the patient was a clinically obese female with a bra size of 44D; the breast shadow was clearly visible during processing (see Figure 7.8); there was no electrocardiogram (ECG) evidence of infarction, and wall movement was normal on gated imaging.

contractility and thickening is good evidence that a defect is due to attenuation. Breast attenuation is relatively easy to recognise, and it rarely presents a significant problem, particularly if gated images are available.

Attenuation correction   Software to correct for attenuation is available, using transmission data either from a line source incorporated in the gantry or from a computed tomography (CT) tube in hybrid scanners. This ought to be the answer to the problems outlined above, and some impressive results can be obtained, with apparent defects disappearing following correction. However, performance is not consistent, and we have not used attenuation correction in clinical practice. One problem is that the correction algorithms can introduce artefacts of their own, the danger being that you lose the reasonably predictable attenuation effects but then have to learn to recognise and allow for an entirely new set of processing artefacts. However, these drawbacks will be overcome, and it may be that by the time this book is published, significant advances will have been made.

Patient movement   Very few patients can keep perfectly still for 20 minutes or more with their arm behind their head, and in a significant minority, the degree of movement is sufficient to cause artefacts in the processed images. Excessive movement should be recognised during inspection of the raw data prior to processing (Figure 7.9).

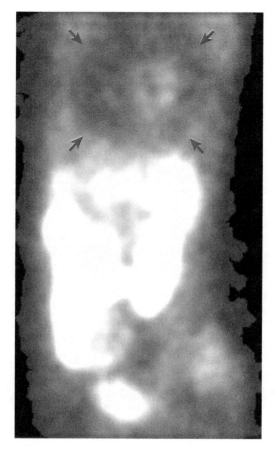

Figure 7.8   This is a single projection from the MPS study of the patient whose processed images are seen in Figure 7.7. Note the large shadow cast by the left breast (arrow). This illustrates the importance of viewing the raw images when reporting MPS studies.

The effect on the processed images depends on the direction of movement, but the most frequent appearance is that of a 'step' in the contour of the ventricle (Figure 7.10) or apparent perfusion defects, usually close to the apex. The only way to avoid being misled by such artefacts is to be aware that excessive movement has occurred, and this requires close communication between the person processing the study and the reporter, when they are not one and the same. Alternatively, the reporter must review the raw data in addition to the processed images and quantitative displays.

Centre of rotation offset   Regular quality assurance should minimise this effect. Typically, centre of rotation offset produces small defects near the apex, not unlike those resulting from patient movement, and elongation or 'smearing' of the apex on the long axis sections.

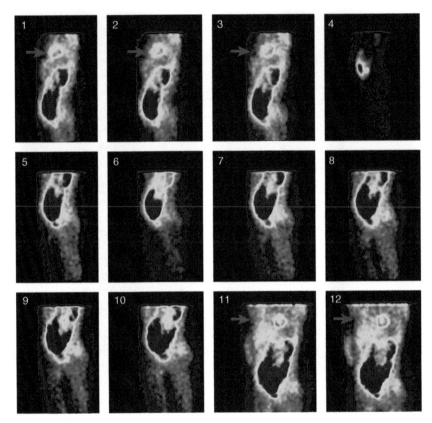

Figure 7.9   Gross patient movement seen on the raw images. Note the upward movement which takes the heart (arrowed at the beginning and end of the sequence) out of the acquisition volume and back in again. This is a particularly bad example, and required rescanning of the patient. Lesser degrees of movement are common, and it is important to recognise it if the resultant abnormalities in the processed images are to be correctly interpreted (see Figure 7.10). Once again, we see the importance of viewing the raw images. In this particular case, the patient had been reaching for her handbag during the acquisition!

Hepatic and gut activity   Although this is not an artefact, it is an unwanted feature of the images, and one which can hinder processing and interpretation. Earlier chapters have outlined the measures taken to minimise the amount of activity beneath the diaphragm, but it is impossible to eliminate completely when using technetium-labelled radiopharmaceuticals (Figure 7.11). It is important to ensure that perceived defects in myocardial uptake are not actually due to scaling problems resulting from high levels of extracardiac activity (Chapter 6).

Misalignment   Again, this is not an artefact, but this time a fault in the processing/display parameters. Failure to align the stress and rest images so that corresponding

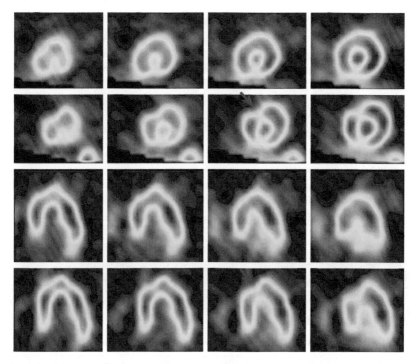

Figure 7.10   Typical 'step' defect produced by patient movement during acquisition (arrow). Usually seen in the anterior wall towards the apex, these defects are fairly easy to recognise, and the raw images should be checked to confirm that movement has occurred. In this case it is the rest images (bottom rows) which are affected. When the movement occurs on the stress images and 'normalises' at rest, it is important to differentiate movement from inducible ischaemia.

sections are presented together can introduce apparent perfusion abnormalities (Figure 7.12). A more subtle example is shown in Chapter 6 (Figure 6.10).

The abnormal perfusion scan

Before describing patterns of abnormality and scan interpretation, it is important to define what we mean by a 'defect'. The images show the *relative* level of activity in each part of the myocardium, with the hottest region being scaled to 100%. We learn to allow for the normal inhomogeneity of uptake (described above), and ascribe any reduction in activity over and above that to a true reduction in perfusion. However, it is possible for a myocardial sector to show *increased* activity, an example being the septal hypertrophy that is occasionally seen in hypertensive patients (Figure 7.13a). Focal hot spots elsewhere in the wall can be due to prominent papillary muscles (Figure 7.13b). It is important to recognise hot spots for

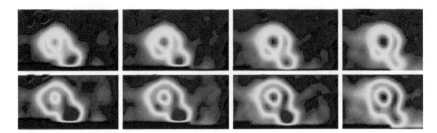

Figure 7.11 High levels of activity beneath the diaphragm producing pseudo defects. In the top row of SA images, no attempt has been made to compensate for the presence of gut activity, and so there are relatively low levels of uptake within the myocardium, particularly the anterior wall. When the images are reprocessed (bottom row) with the hottest part of the left ventricle scaled to maximum, the cardiac activity can be seen to be normal.

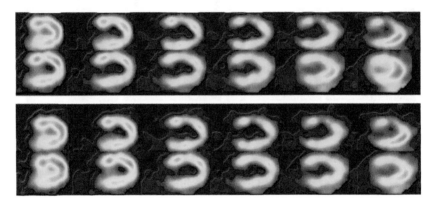

Figure 7.12 VLA images illustrating the effect of misalignment. In the top (misaligned) pair of sequences (stress above, rest below), the two frames at the right-hand end appear to show reversibility in the anterior wall. On the lower two sequences following realignment, that is no longer the case.

what they are, because they will result in a relative reduction in uptake elsewhere which can be interpreted as a defect, and when processing the images the scaling must be adjusted to minimise this effect (see Chapter 6). Similarly, balanced three-vessel disease can give rise to an apparently normal scan when the blood flow in each vessel is equally poor. Fortunately, this happens relatively infrequently, and in three-vessel disease, one vessel is usually significantly more affected than the others, so that a relative defect is still produced. However, the extent of the disease may consequently be underestimated, and this is where secondary signs of extensive disease become important (see 'Other prognostic indicators' below). Semiquantitative analysis using suitably scaled polar (bull's-eye) plots can also be helpful in this situation (see Chapter 6).

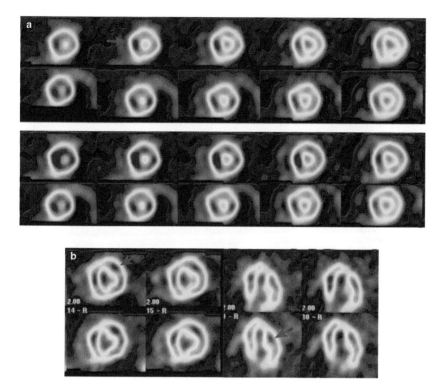

Figure 7.13 (a) SA views in a patient with left ventricular hypertrophy, showing the hot spot in the septum (arrow) which is often seen in these patients, and which can result in an apparent reduction in activity elsewhere in the ventricle. In the lower pair of sequences, the images have been rescaled to the lateral wall, which results in a more normal appearance of the myocardium, but with oversaturation of the hot septum. (b) SA (left) and HLA (right) images showing a hot spot in the lateral wall (arrow) attributable to a papillary muscle.

Key point   It is all relative

MPS image illustrate relative, not absolute, perfusion. This has implications for interpretation:

- Three-vessel disease can produce a normal scan if perfusion is equally poor in each vascular territory. Secondary indicators of extensive disease then become important
- Physiological or pathological hot spots in the myocardium will result in apparent reductions in perfusion elsewhere, and these must be differentiated from genuine perfusion defects

Defects can be graded for severity in a number of ways, the simplest being a three-point scale of mild, moderate and severe. A mild defect is defined as one showing

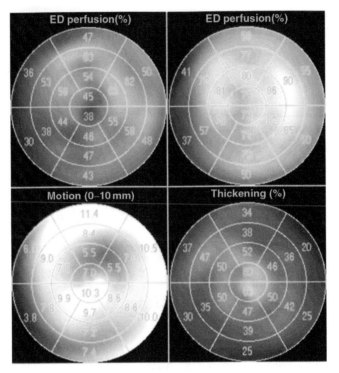

Figure 7.14 Diagram showing the segments used for numerical scoring of defects.

reduced activity but no obvious reduction in thickness of the myocardium; a moderate defect as a more marked reduction in activity associated with apparent thinning of the myocardium; and a severe defect as one showing levels of uptake comparable with background. These are scored from 1 to 3 (normal perfusion being 0). Clearly this is all very subjective, and the apparent severity of defects can be influenced by a number of factors other than the actual level of perfusion. Scoring systems divide the myocardium into anything from 9 to 20 segments (Figure 7.14), each of which is evaluated separately. The segmental scores are added to give a summed stress score (SSS) and a summed rest score (SRS). Subtracting the SRS from the SSS gives the summed difference score (SDS), thus giving a semiquantitative index of the at-risk myocardium. Some reporters undertake this numerical analysis for all scans; others, this author included, assess the extent and severity of the perfusion defects by eye, and then give an opinion as to their prognostic significance and the need for further investigation (see also 'Quantitative or qualitative?' above). However, the more formal analysis is of value in the detection of hibernating myocardium (see 'Assessment of viability' below). Finally in this introductory section there is a reminder of the potential for confusion around the description of defects as 'reversible' or 'inducible'. In this chapter, we will use the word reversible, because most people do, and we all know what we mean by it.

Key point   Reversible or inducible?

Defects are not reversed by rest; they are actively induced by stress, due to an increase in the oxygen demands of the myocardium and consequent dilatation of those coronary artery branches able to do so

However, the description of defects as 'reversible' or irreversible' is now enshrined in common usage, and regardless of its semantic imprecision, we will stick to that form of words

---

Single perfusion defects

By 'single' we mean a well-defined defect, fixed or reversible, usually corresponding to the whole or part of one of the three main vascular territories (although these can be variable – see above). Despite what we have said about the variability of the coronary vascular supply, many single defects correspond convincingly to the areas of myocardium subtended by the right coronary artery (RCA), the left main stem (LMS), the left anterior descending (LAD), and the circumflex (Cx) arteries (Figure 7.1c). Examples of some focal defects are shown in Figure 7.15.

Multiple vessel disease

Defects which are too extensive or numerous to be the result of a single anatomical lesion may be attributed to multivessel disease, although care should be taken when it is simply the position of a defect that implies lesions in more than one vessel, since it may be the result of normal anatomical variation. Our practice with more extensive abnormalities is to describe their distribution rather than listing the arterial territories potentially involved. This also allows for the fact that the perfusion images may underestimate the extent of disease when more than one vessel is involved (see above). It is the size and severity of the defects, rather than the number of vessels involved, which is important in prognosis, although these parameters are clearly related. The 'Other prognostic indicators' mentioned below can be important clues to the presence of more extensive or severe disease than may be apparent from the perfusion images alone.

Fixed or reversible?

Sometimes, defects on stress images clearly normalise completely at rest. More often though, there is only partial recovery, which begs the question of how much

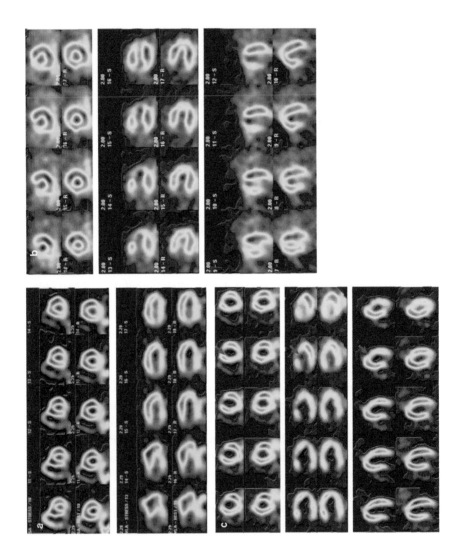

Figure 7.15
(Continued)

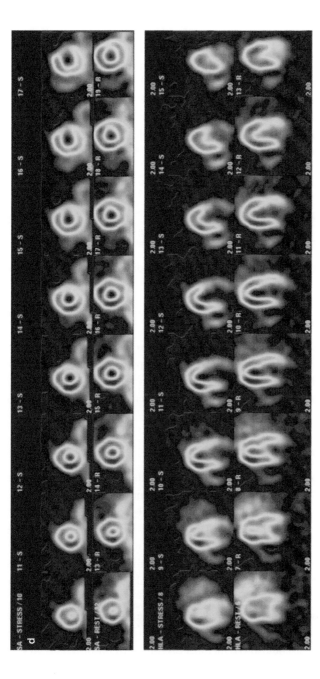

Figure 7.15 (a) Inferior wall defect due to right coronary disease. Note the large right ventricle (RV). (b) Reversible defects in the LAD territory: note the involvement of the apex, anterior wall and septum. (c) Typical defect in the anterolateral wall of the left ventricle (LV) due to a lesion in the diagonal branch of the LAD (arrows). (d) Reversible defect involving the lateral wall of the LV in a patient with isolated stenosis of the circumflex artery. However, defects will often not relate clearly to a particular vascular territory, and the areas of myocardium subtended by the individual vessels can vary significantly between patients. It is therefore often better to report the position and extent of myocardial involvement rather than attributing defects to specific vessels (see text).

change there has to be before the defect is classified as reversible. Attempts have been made to quantify this, and software such as QPS (quantitative perfusion SPECT) will highlight defects which are considered to qualify. These quantitative approaches offer some assistance to inexperienced reporters, but with the passage of time you acquire a 'feel' for what represents genuine reversibility, and this is not based simply on an analysis of the activity levels in the involved segment at stress and rest – it will also take into account the clinical history and other information such as the sex, height and weight of the patient. For example, the same partially reversible defect in the anterior wall of the left ventricle will be interpreted differently in a 100-kg female patient with a low clinical probability of disease and a slim male with a known 70% stenosis of the LAD and a convincing clinical history.

Other prognostic indicators

Impaired left ventricular function

This is the most important supplementary indicator of poor prognosis, and is covered in 'Functional indices' below.

Prominent right ventricular uptake

An apparent increase in right ventricular uptake can be a reflection of a generalised *reduction* in left ventricular activity. This is seen in patients with severe three-vessel disease, although in the absence of other signs of left ventricular hypoperfusion, it is far more likely to be due to right ventricular hypertrophy (see 'Other patterns to recognise' below).

Transient ischaemic dilatation

This description of an apparent increase in size of the ventricular cavity at stress as compared to rest (Figure 7.16) is probably a misnomer. Although there are cases where true dilatation occurs, transient ischaemic dilatation (TID) is probably more often due to widespread subendocardial ischaemia, implying multivessel disease – hence the negative prognostic implications of the sign. When perfusion is clearly abnormal, there is no problem in reporting TID, but it can be seen in the presence of normal or near-normal perfusion images. Here it takes a slightly bolder reporter to believe the evidence of his or her eyes, but it can be the only indicator of balanced three-vessel disease (see above). In this situation, the clinical context will be important in deciding how much weight to give to TID, as will the magnitude of the discrepancy in size. You should also remember to ensure that the difference in size is not due to an error in processing, with a different zoom factor applied to the stress and rest images, or to the acquisition of the two datasets on different technical settings, or different patient geometry.

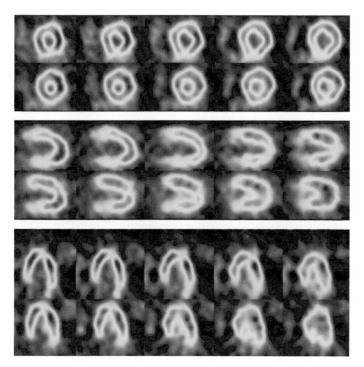

Figure 7.16   Transient ischaemic dilatation (TID) in a patient with proven three-vessel disease. SA views showing the increased size of the left ventricular cavity on the stress (top) images compared to those at rest. While this can be due to genuine changes in volume, it should be remembered that although the radiopharmaceutical is injected at peak stress, the patient is usually well into the recovery phase by the time images are acquired. It is likely that this appearance is actually due to widespread subendocardial ischaemia, which is not present when injection is performed at rest, and that the increase in volume is therefore more apparent than real. TID can be the only indicator of extensive ischaemia in those (thankfully rare) patients with perfectly balanced three-vessel disease. In this case, the abnormalities are not evenly distributed, and there is more severe involvement of the inferior and, to a lesser extent, the anterior walls, where there is evidence of reversibility.

Increased lung uptake

This parameter was described in relation to thallium scanning, and has been demonstrated to occur in patients with a failing left ventricle, and a consequent increase in pulmonary venous pressure. It therefore has the same prognostic implications as an abnormal gated scan (see 'Interpreting and reporting the gated scan' below). Although there have been descriptions of a similar appearance using technetium agents, there is no agreement on its significance at the time of writing, and so this is really a sign that can only be relied upon when using thallium, when a lung/cardiac count ratio of >50% is often taken as the threshold for abnormality.

Key point   LBBB

Remember that in left bundle branch block:

- Relative defects may be seen in the septum in the absence of ischaemia
- These may be accentuated by tachycardia
- Adenosine is therefore the stressor of choice, due to its lack of inotropic effects

Other patterns to recognise

Left bundle branch block

As conduction defects make ECG interpretation difficult, standard exercise testing in the diagnosis of ischaemic heart disease is not possible, and MPS is often requested as an alternative in these patients. So it is unfortunate that the presence of left bundle branch block (LBBB) can be the cause of abnormalities in MPS images in the absence of ischaemia. Typically, there is reduced uptake in the septum, which should be fixed (Figure 7.17). However, it is important to note that the relative defect can be accentuated by tachycardia, and so any form of stress which increases the heart rate (treadmill exercise or dobutamine) may result in a defect which appears to be at least partially reversible. Adenosine is therefore the stressor of choice, due to its lack of inotropic effects. Even when adenosine is used, LBBB may make interpretation difficult if abnormalities are confined to the LAD territory, especially if the defect due to the conduction abnormality encroaches on the anterior wall. However, MPS is still useful in these patients, as any convincing reversibility in the septum/anterior wall, or evidence of ischaemia elsewhere, will be indicators that further investigation is needed, usually angiography. Equally, the presence of a fixed reduction in septal uptake in the absence of any other abnormality provides reassurance that there is no significant inducible ischaemia underlying the conduction abnormality.

Left ventricular hypertrophy

MPS is not used to diagnose left ventricular hypertrophy (LVH), but it is important to recognise the effects it may have on the appearance of the scan images. Not surprisingly, the gated images may demonstrate increased thickness of the ventricular wall and a reduced cavity size (Figure 7.18a). Sometimes this can result in a relative hot spot in the septum (Figure 7.13a). Gated imaging will often reveal a small ventricular volume and unusually high ejection fraction, and wall thickening may be apparent when both the inner and outer contours of the ventricular wall are displayed (Figure 7.18b). Having said all that, it is not unusual to see normal MPS images in patients with proven LVH.

Right ventricular abnormalities

Dilatation and/or hypertrophy of the right ventricle will result in unusually prominent right ventricular activity on the perfusion images. This may be seen in association with

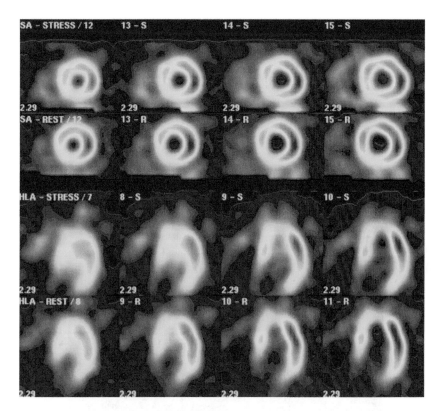

Figure 7.17 Left bundle branch block. Note the reduced uptake in the septum and anteroseptal regions. Typically, the defects are fixed, as in this case. However, stress techniques which result in increased heart rate can produce defects which are worse during stress, mimicking inducible ischaemia. Adenosine is therefore the stressor of choice in these patients. In this patient, there is also a fixed inferior defect, which was the result of previous infarction.

an enlarged left ventricle in patients with dilated cardiomyopathy (Figure 7.19a), and where it is an isolated finding, it will often be the result of chronic respiratory disease (Figure 7.19b).

INTERPRETING AND REPORTING THE GATED SCAN

Introduction

Gated imaging provides information on regional wall movement, wall thickening and numerical measures of function, of which the most frequently used is the ejection fraction. Most software packages produce a final report screen which portrays

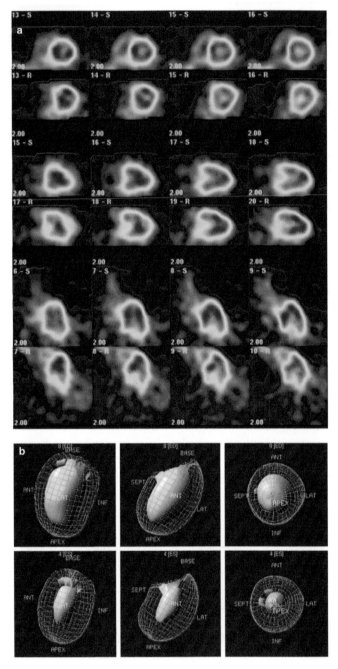

Figure 7.18 (a) Left ventricular hypertrophy (see also Figure 7.13a). Note the thick wall and small ventricular cavity, which appears to be almost obliterated. (b) Gated imaging in the same patient – diastolic phase (upper row) and systolic (lower). This highlights the thickening of the wall (blue contour = inner surface of ventricle, brown mesh = outer surface). The end diastolic volume was measured as 48 cm^3, and the ejection fraction was 70%.

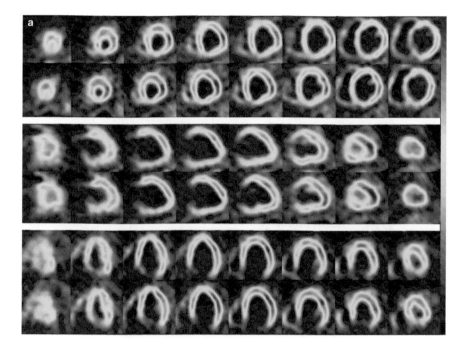

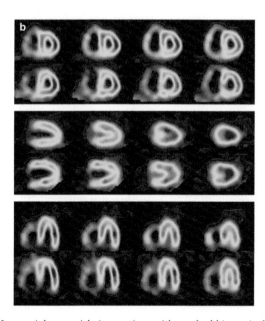

Figure 7.19   (a) Large right ventricle in a patient with marked biventricular dilatation. Best appreciated on the basal SA sections (top right). (b) Prominent RV activity in a patient with chronic pulmonary disease and a normal sized left ventricle. In this case, note the straight septum, giving the LV a 'D' shape, an appearance seen in patients with pulmonary hypertension and RV overload.

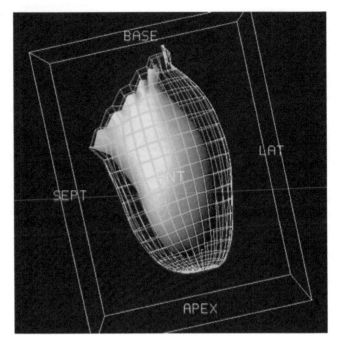

Figure 7.20   Gated display showing the end diastolic (green mesh) and the end systolic (solid blue) contours of the ventricle. The ventricle can be 'spun' to show the different walls in profile (Figure 7.18b), and so assess wall movement, which in this case is normal.

these data in some form, often as a numerical map. In routine reporting, this functional information serves two main purposes: to help to differentiate between fixed defects due to ischaemia and those due to attenuation, and to give an overall indication of ventricular function for prognostic purposes (see Chapter 8).

In assessing the gated images, it is important to remember that they were derived from the same data that you have already seen presented as perfusion images. If those were degraded by attenuation, patient movement, the presence of high levels of activity in the liver or gut, or all of these, then it is unreasonable to expect the software to produce flawless gated images. The old computing aphorism of 'rubbish in, rubbish out' again applies here, and so local abnormalities of wall movement or unexpectedly low values for the ejection fraction must be interpreted with caution in these circumstances.

Wall motion

This is probably best appreciated on the cine display, which can be viewed from several different directions in order to demonstrate each wall of the ventricle (Figure 7.20). Software packages will produce a map of wall movement, assigning a numerical value to the degree of movement during systole for each area, often on

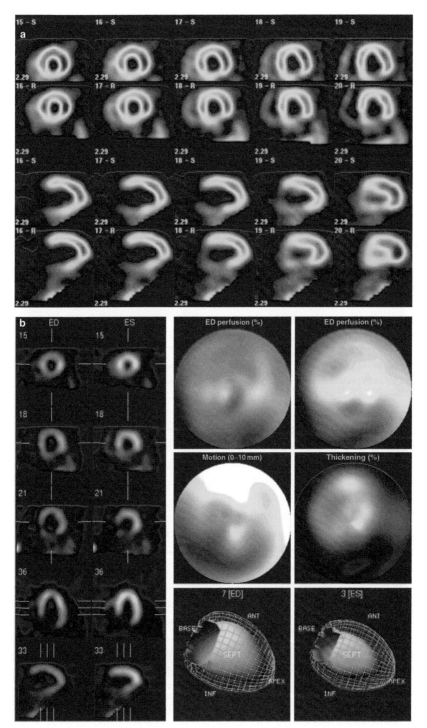

Figure 7.21 (a) There is a fixed inferior defect in this patient with a well-documented previous infarct. (b) Image from the gated acquisition on the same patient. Wall movement was

Figure 7.21   (Continued)

normal, but the slices on the left, at end diastole and end systole, show some impairment of wall thickening. Note the increase in brightness between the end-diastolic and end-systolic slices in those areas with relatively normal thickening (i.e. everywhere except the inferior wall). This is also indicated in the polar representation of thickening (middle image in right-hand column).

a scale of 0 (normal) to 5 (dyskinetic). It is also possible to view the images on which these maps are based, presented as orthogonal slices moving in real time (Figure 7.21b). The septum typically shows less movement than the free walls of the ventricle, and it is important to note that this disparity is more marked in patients who have undergone previous open heart surgery. In these postoperative patients there may be gross reductions in septal wall movement in the absence of significant ischaemia: another reason to insist on accurate clinical information before attempting to interpret scans. There also tends to be a reduction in wall movement at the base of the heart, particularly inferiorly, and too much importance should not be attributed to this in the absence of abnormality elsewhere.

Key point   Postoperative appearances

Septal hypokinesia or akinesia is frequently seen following cardiac surgery, and should not be interpreted as evidence of functional abnormality

---

Knowledge of wall motion is most often of use in assessing the significance of fixed perfusion defects. If the affected segment of myocardium moves normally, the assumption will be that the defect is the result of attenuation. Where this is the case, the reporter's suspicions will usually already have been aroused by the fact that there is no history or ECG evidence of infarction, and by the knowledge that the patient's physique is of a type likely to result in excessive attenuation. Even so, it is very reassuring to see the region in question contracting normally.

What is slightly disconcerting is the number of occasions on which a patient with a history of infarction underpinned by good clinical, biochemical and electrocardiographic evidence and a fixed perfusion defect in the right place turns out to have reasonably good movement of the relevant segment on gated imaging (Figure 7.21a and b). This may reflect the presence of a partial rather than full-thickness infarct, but also the fact that these tend to be clinically stable outpatients with mature infarcts and good surrounding contractility, which 'pulls' the infarcted segment inwards during systole. In any case, this observation does not usually present a clinical problem, as the referring cardiologist will be more interested in the presence or absence of ischaemia elsewhere in the myocardium than in the behaviour of a known infarct. More importantly, it does not undermine the negative predictive value of normal wall movement in those patients with a low probability of infarction described in the previous paragraph.

What about patients with a low probability of infarction and a fixed defect, initially thought to be due to attenuation, who unexpectedly prove to have impaired wall movement on gated imaging? As with all clinical testing, the predictive value of a positive test in such a patient group will be relatively low, and the weight to be attached to the finding will depend on:

- the degree of abnormality demonstrated
- the clinical context
- the presence or absence of abnormalities elsewhere in the myocardium
- the technical quality of the study.

If there is clear evidence of ischaemia elsewhere, this will usually be the driver for management decisions, and so uncertainty over the relevance of the hypokinetic segment may not be a problem clinically. In these cases, the 'fixed' defect may actually represent hibernating myocardium (see 'Assessment of viability' below), and careful semiquantitative analysis may reveal that there is actually some relative improvement in perfusion which was not so apparent on purely visual examination. Where the fixed defect with impaired movement is the only abnormality, the clinically important decision to be made is not so much between infarction and attenuation as between attenuation and hibernation. This relatively unusual situation is where careful consideration of the bullet points above becomes important, as every case is different. Where it is not immediately apparent that the abnormality can be explained by attenuation or other technical factors, the significance of the findings should be discussed with the relevant cardiologist.

Wall thickening

Wall thickening, like wall movement, is an indicator of normally functioning myocardium. Software packages present the data in a similar format to that for wall movement, with maps showing numerical values for systolic thickening and moving displays of orthogonal sections through the ventricle (Figure 7.21b). When viewing the real-time display, it is important to appreciate that what you are looking for is not the actual thickening of the wall, but an increase in its brightness, as more activity is concentrated into a smaller area. There are few data concerning the significance of thickening as an independent variable – in routine reporting it is usually considered along with wall movement. However, where there is doubt over the relevance of wall motion abnormalities, the degree of wall thickening can be helpful, and it is also important in assessing the response to low-dose dobutamine (below).

Functional indices

The numerical indices most often quoted are the left ventricular ejection fraction (LVEF) and ventricular volume. Here it is important to ensure that the software used is properly calibrated to the gamma camera with respect to variables such as pixel size, in order to ensure that accurate results are produced. It is equally important to then develop a normal range of values based on your own equipment and patient population. Knowledge of the LVEF and ventricular volume is clearly of importance in its own right as a marker of cardiac function, but it has additional prognostic significance in relation to MPS. Impaired function increases the prognostic significance of any ischaemia demonstrated on the perfusion images, and this should be reflected in the report.

Gated imaging also produces a number of other indices, largely those involved in the assessment of diastolic dysfunction, usually in patients suffering from heart failure. However, MPS packages may use as few as eight frames for the gated acquisition, and a time/activity curve derived from just eight data points does not allow detailed analysis of the dynamics of ventricular filling and emptying. Consequently, echocardiography tends to be the method of choice in this role, and in routine MPS reporting it is unusual to consider parameters other than LVEF and ventricular volume.

Gated imaging under stress

We routinely perform gated imaging at the time of the rest study, on the assumption that perfusion defects are likely to be at a minimum, and the quality of the gated study will consequently be optimised. Even if the gating is performed after the stress injection, the patient will still be at rest when the imaging is carried out, and so the parameters measured will reflect the situation at rest. It can be useful to measure function during stress, but the patient must be subjected to that stress, physical or pharmacological, at the time of the acquisition. Physical stress is difficult to achieve without a couch-mounted bicycle ergometer, but low-dose dobutamine studies can be useful (see 'Assessment of viability' below).

ASSESSMENT OF VIABILITY

Definitions

Purists argue with the use of the term 'viability', but it is widely accepted, and so it is important to understand what is meant by it. Viability is really a clinical concept, reflecting the fact that some patients with chronic ischaemic heart disease manifested on MPS as fixed perfusion defects with impaired contractility nevertheless demonstrate functional recovery following revascularization. Strictly speaking, this should not happen, because:

fixed perfusion defect + impaired contractility = infarction

So there is clearly more to interpreting a perfusion scan than simply recognizing defects and characterizing them as fixed or reversible. Understanding what is happening in these areas of apparently dead but actually 'viable' myocardium requires the introduction of the concepts of myocardial stunning and hibernation. A lot of work has been done to determine the cellular processes underlying these states, but brief working definitions are as follows.

Stunning

This refers to impairment of myocardial function due to an episode of ischaemia which persists following the restoration of blood flow. The duration of the stunning effect depends to some extent on the degree and duration of the ischaemic episode, but recovery will eventually occur, provided that normal blood flow is maintained. Stunning therefore manifests itself on MPS as areas of reduced contractility with normal perfusion.

Hibernation

Hibernating myocardium is chronically ischaemic with reduced motility, and in some cases this may be the result of repetitive stunning. Hibernation can be viewed as a protective mechanism, whereby the reduced contractility allows myocytes to maintain their cellular integrity by matching their oxygen demand to the chronically reduced blood flow. Hibernating myocardium will consequently result in fixed perfusion defects with impaired contractility on MPS.

It is therefore important to differentiate patients with chronic ischaemic heart disease and left ventricular dysfunction who would benefit from reperfusion from those with irreversible impairment of function, and several nuclear cardiology techniques have been used to assess myocardial viability.

Thallium imaging and viability

Thallium stress protocols involving re-injection at rest, or rest imaging followed by a redistribution study, have been shown to have good predictive value for the detection of viable myocardium. However, most centres taking up MPS will be using technetium-labelled agents, in view of their many advantages over thallium, so this will not be considered in more detail.

Technetium agents and viability

Unlike thallium, tetrofosmin and sestamibi do not redistribute. This is a potential disadvantage in the recognition of hibernation, since a rest injection of Tc agent will still show reduced perfusion. However, quantitative or semiquantitative assessment of uptake following rest injection combined with nitrate administration has been shown to have similar accuracy in the assessment of viability to the thallium protocols mentioned above.

Gated imaging with low-dose dobutamine

This is the scintigraphic equivalent of dobutamine echocardiography, and aims to demonstrate contractile reserve in hibernating myocardium. It relies on the fact that in hibernating myocardium, the reduction in contractility is due at least partly to the protective downregulation in metabolism, and not just to the reduced blood flow. Low-level inotropic stimulation can therefore produce an initial improvement in contractility before increased oxygen demands, which cannot be met due to the restricted blood flow, produce an adverse effect on function. Reporting is fairly straightforward: the standard gated acquisition is performed with and without low-dose (5 μg/kg/min) dobutamine infusion. Wall movement and thickening of the affected area of myocardium, and the LVEF, are compared. Visual improvement in contractility, hopefully backed up by the software's quantitative assessment, is an indication of viability, as is an improvement in LVEF of 5% or more.

Fluorodeoxyglucose imaging

Fluorodeoxyglucose (FDG) uptake is an indicator of continuing active metabolism, and therefore a good marker of viability. Imaging can be performed on standard gamma cameras fitted with high energy collimators, to cope with the 511-keV photons resulting from the annihilation events when the positrons emitted by ^{18}F meet an electron. However, 'proper' positron emission tomography (PET) using a dedicated PET scanner is the method of choice for imaging with FDG, but until this equipment is more widely available, cardiac imaging will probably have to take second place to the proven indications for PET in the diagnosis and follow-up of malignant disease. As FDG imaging is unlikely to be available to departments setting up an MPS service, it will not be considered further.

Cardiac magnetic resonance imaging

This is another technique showing considerable promise in this area, but it is outside the scope of this book.

CONCLUSION

Surprisingly few texts on MPS (or on radiology in general) actually address the issue of how to report scans, and this chapter has been an attempt to cover the essentials for those just starting an MPS service. However, as with most imaging techniques, the reporting of scans is as much an art as a science, and there is no substitute for experience. The key messages to take away are: do not over-report scans, and try to involve your cardiology colleagues, especially during the early days of the new service.

8

Myocardial perfusion scintigraphy in clinical management

INTRODUCTION

This final chapter is not intended to be an exhaustive account of the clinical applications of nuclear cardiology and myocardial perfusion scintigraphy (MPS) in particular. This information may be found in the comprehensive texts and reviews[1] devoted to the subject and the detailed guidelines published by the relevant societies.[2,3] Here we aim to provide an overview of what the cardiologist wants from nuclear cardiology and what we in nuclear cardiology offer the cardiologist. There is an intentional clinical bias, discussing the patient groups in whom myocardial perfusion imaging is of particular diagnostic and prognostic value. We include several relevant clinical cases to highlight some of the points raised. Novel nuclear cardiological techniques (for example cardiac neurotransmitter, receptor and molecular imaging) are currently more research-orientated, not widely available in the UK, and beyond the remit of this practical handbook.

WHAT THE CARDIOLOGIST WANTS FROM THE REPORT

The perfusion scan report is the important information returned to the referring cardiologist that guides patient management. Clearly the quality of the report reflects not only on the interpreting cardiologist or radiologist but also on the quality and efficiency of your department. It is of no surprise that both your report and the service you provide also affect how your referring cardiologists view the field of nuclear cardiology. A well run, efficient service with a short waiting list which provides accurate and clear reports is unlikely to attract the rather derogatory title of 'unclear cardiology'.

The clarity of the report is vital. Cardiologists do not want to receive a report scattered with 'suggestive of', 'possible', 'equivocal' or 'of unknown significance'. Nor do they want over-reporting of scans which will increase the false positive rate of the test. Faced with an ambiguous report most cardiologists I know will send the patient for an angiogram, and if they find disease-free coronary arteries, they will lose faith in nuclear cardiology and stop referring appropriate patients. Not only is this expensive, but it also exposes the patient to the unnecessary risk of an invasive test. If you can deliver a timely service with accurate reports, angiography can be targeted at those with a greater clinical risk, and when you have impressed your colleagues they hopefully should and will start accessing your service more often. We have witnessed this happening since we managed to increase our activity and get our waiting times down.

Frustratingly there will be times where it is not possible to answer confidently the question posed when issuing a report. This often occurs when patients move, bowel gets in the way, or gating is not possible due to arrhythmias. In these instances the clinical judgement of the reporter (if in possession of sufficient information) and the referrer is important. We find as reporters that it is preferable to be honest (and humble) in these situations and explain why it is not possible to be definitive, rather than issue a 'possibly' type of report. Depending on the degree of clinical suspicion and risk stratification of the patient it is not always necessary to go on to do another test.

Nuclear cardiology in the UK has of course been its own worst enemy. Where waiting times are very long, MPS is devalued as a useful test. Waiting a year to find out if an exercise test is falsely positive is unacceptable, and consequently MPS will not be requested and the patient will be subjected to the risks of angiography. Having to wait an age to assess the functional significance of a coronary artery stenosis is equally inappropriate. Inevitably the interventionalist will succumb to the urge to intervene, and blow up a balloon to open the artery whether it is needed or not!

As mentioned above we have noted that as waiting times have come down in our department there has been an increase in the appropriate use of MPS. If the waiting time does extend to 12 months, those attending your department are likely to be low-risk patients, or those that the cardiologist does not want to subject to angiography. It is frustrating to report a whole pile of normal scans! With shorter waits our interventional cardiologists are using our department to assess the need for revascularization post-angiography, and indeed prior to angiography to investigate symptoms post-revascularization.

To continue to develop and thrive, nuclear cardiology needs to continue to aim for the shortest possible waiting times while maintaining the quality of studies and reports. A high quality report containing maximum clinical information and answering the referrer's question (if they have asked one!) will help to ensure continued and increased referrals. This is certainly a challenge, particularly with the 18-week referral-to-treatment government target about to kick in. However, using MPS early in the investigation strategy is known to be cost-effective,[4] and we should not forget to keep reminding our cardiology colleagues of this fact.

WHAT NUCLEAR CARDIOLOGY NEEDS FROM THE REFERRAL

It is all too easy for colleagues in cardiology to be cynical of 'unclear cardiology' if we fall into the trap of providing unhelpful reports and sit on the fence rather than

Table 8.1 National Institute for Health and Clinical Excellence (NICE) Technology Appraisal 73 (November 2003):[5] 'Myocardial perfusion scintigraphy for the diagnosis and management of angina and myocardial infarction'

The conclusion reached by NICE was that for this purpose MPS is both clinically effective and cost-effective. Their recommendations were that MPS should be used in the following situations:

- As the initial diagnostic test for patients with suspected coronary artery disease (CAD) where an exercise test poses particular problems including conduction defects and resting ECG abnormalities, those incapable of exercise, women and those with diabetes

- As an investigation for diagnosing suspected CAD in people with a lower likelihood of CAD

- As an investigation in patients with symptoms following myocardial infarction or coronary revascularization (CABG and PCI)

NICE suggested that a level of MPS provision should be 4000 studies per million population per year and that the current activity level fell far short of this at 1200. They also indicated that suitable waiting times should be a maximum of 6 weeks for a routine study and 1 week for an urgent scan

---

CABG, coronary artery bypass grafting; PCI, percutaneous coronary intervention.

giving them something definitive. Equally the referring cardiologist will get the most from the nuclear cardiology department if they give us all the relevant information. A referral that states 'single vessel disease, 80% stenosis, assess significance' is a typical case in point. Are they just trying us out for our accuracy? The name of the vessel might be a start. Are they just lazy at filling in the form? If the request is from an interventionalist why have they not blown up a balloon already – what else is going on? It is of course entirely reasonable to ask for more information from the referring clinician.

Why do referrers think that we will have more success with the morbidly obese patient who is too heavy for the treadmill or the catheterization laboratory table and who could not have a stress echo due to lack of an acoustic window? It is up to you to work closely with your cardiologists and continue to educate them. Having a cardiology trainee attached to the department is a good opportunity to spread the word about using the department appropriately. The rapid-access chest pain clinic has led to the expectation among many that if the patient cannot exercise then they need an alternative test, but history, examination and assessment of risk need to come first. Equally we should work with the chest pain clinic to avoid duplication of tests by offering MPS as a first line investigation where appropriate (Table 8.1). Once again this depends on short waiting times, as the treadmill is readily available in the clinic and inevitably becomes the chosen test by default even when not necessarily appropriate.

WHY SHOULD THE CARDIOLOGIST CHOOSE MYOCARDIAL PERFUSION SCINTIGRAPHY?

We know that MPS is a valuable diagnostic and prognostic tool available to the cardiologist managing patients with suspected or documented coronary artery disease. The risk of cardiac death or non-fatal myocardial infarction predicted by a normal MPS study is 0.6% a year for 5 years.[6] This prognostic value is independent even of the results of coronary angiography, and patients with other markers of poor prognosis (including ST depression with exercise) still have a good prognosis if they have a normal MPS.[2] This clearly has significant implications for the management and follow-up of patients.

The National Institute for Health and Clinical Excellence (NICE) have also made recommendations on the use of MPS[5] (see Table 8.1 for summary), though for this to be deliverable there needs to be increased provision of nuclear cardiology in the UK. Although MPS features in most clinical guidelines for the investigation and treatment of angina,[7,8] MPS activity in the UK is considerably lower that in the US and Europe.[9] This is reflected in the number of scans performed compared to coronary revascularization rates. It is only with increased provision that more cardiologists will refer patients to your department.

So we know that MPS is of value in all patients, but it is of particular benefit in those in whom the exercise test is unhelpful, either because of resting electrocardiogram (ECG) abnormalities, in women, in patients with diabetes or hypertension, and in those who are unable to achieve their target heart rate. MPS is also of value in assessing acute chest pain and in guiding revascularization (coronary artery bypass grafting (CABG) or percutaneous coronary intervention (PCI)) by determining the haemodynamic significance of observed coronary lesions. There is also a role for MPS in assessing the adequacy of revascularization. Post-myocardial infarction, MPS can determine the likelihood of future coronary events and can risk-stratify patients with vascular disease who are scheduled to undergo non-cardiac surgery. MPS has a part to play in the evaluation of myocardial viability and hibernation, particularly with reference to planned revascularization, and is also useful in the assessment of left ventricular function, for example in monitoring the effects of cytotoxic chemotherapy or measuring the ejection fraction in patients who may fulfil the criteria for defibrillator implantation.[2,10,11]

Clinical case A

A 50-year-old male smoker is referred to the cardiology clinic with exertional chest pain and breathlessness. Clinical examination is normal but his resting ECG shows right bundle branch block (Figure 8.1a)

A recent ankle injury makes exercise testing impossible so adenosine stress MPS is performed. The scan (Figure 8.1b) shows normal myocardial perfusion at both stress (upper row) and rest (lower row)

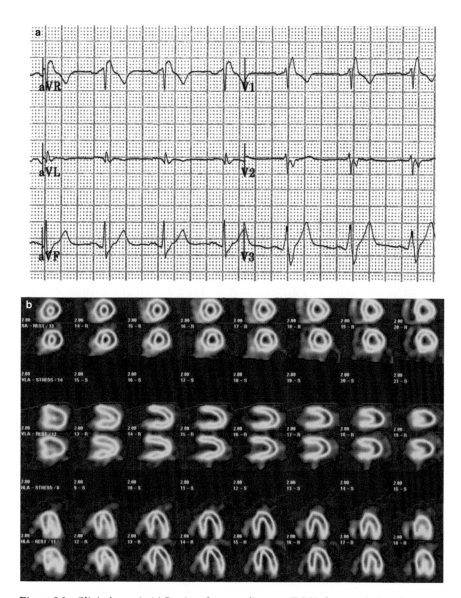

Figure 8.1 Clinical case A. (a) Resting electrocardiogram (ECG) shows right bundle branch block. (b) Normal myocardial perfusion at both stress (upper row) and rest (lower row).

WHY THE CARDIOLOGIST SHOULD CHOOSE MYOCARDIAL PERFUSION SCINTIGRAPHY: COST-EFFECTIVENESS

In the current economic environment of the National Health Service (NHS) the importance of the cost-effectiveness of MPS should not be underestimated. Delivery of the 18-week target also favours using MPS earlier in the diagnostic pathway (providing you can offer easy access to your service). We know from the EMPIRE study (Economics of Myocardial Perfusion Imaging in Europe) that using MPS in the diagnostic pathway costs less and is as effective as those diagnostic strategies which use other investigations.[4] This applies to the cost of both diagnosis and patient management for the next 2 years. The high sensitivity of MPS avoids the need for a secondary test, which is not the case if a less accurate primary test is used (for example an exercise treadmill test in the hypertensive patient producing a possible false positive result). Early and accurate diagnosis, as a result of the high sensitivity of MPS, reduces the likelihood of future cardiac events, with a consequent saving in treatment costs. The need for additional investigations, particularly angiography, is reduced, and not only is this appropriate use of resources but it is also of benefit to the patient in reducing the time taken to achieve diagnosis and treatment.

The prognostic information provided by MPS is an added advantage, and means that appropriate patients – those with the most to gain from treatment – can be selected for further intervention. It has been demonstrated that with respect to life-years saved, increased use of MPS not only improves the cost-effectiveness of treatment but also improves patient outcomes. This is particularly the case in women, patients with diabetes and the elderly.[12]

Women and MPS

Cardiovascular disease remains the leading cause of death among women. Women who have a myocardial infarction (MI) are more likely to die or suffer a further MI during the following year than are men.[13] Women's symptoms are clinically more difficult to evaluate: angina is often atypical. Although exercise testing is the screening test most frequently used to detect coronary artery disease it has a lower diagnostic accuracy in women than in men, due largely to a higher false positive rate.[14] Also, women often have a lower exercise capacity than men and are unable to exercise for a sufficient duration to attain their target heart rate. Premenopausal women have a high prevalence of non-cardiac chest pain.

All these factors mean that not only is coronary artery disease (CAD) underdiagnosed in women but they are also often referred for coronary angiography on the basis of an inconclusive or false positive test. In women being investigated for chest pain, when coronary angiography is performed, it is common to find disease-free coronary arteries.[15]

For all levels of exercise, stress technetium single photon emission computed tomography (SPECT) imaging techniques have been shown to be more accurate in diagnosing CAD than exercise testing alone. Furthermore, the diagnostic accuracy of pharmacological stress MPS is also high (regardless of the pharmacological agent used), and should be used in women unable to exercise.[16] Previously there have been limitations as a result of anterior attenuation artefacts in women (breast attenuation), but these have been largely overcome with the use of gated SPECT imaging and attenuation correction.

In the UK, NICE recommends the use of MPS as a first line investigative test in women with suspected coronary artery disease (Table 8.1). This strategy avoids the unnecessary risks of angiography and is cost-effective. For the same reasons, MPS is of proven value in investigating women with known coronary artery disease.

Clinical case B

A 54-year-old woman with exertional breathlessness, chest tightness, and hypertension is referred to the chest pain clinic. Examination and resting ECG are normal and she completes 3 minutes 50 seconds of a Bruce protocol treadmill test, stopping because of breathlessness. There is inferolateral ST depression with a maximum of 1.5 mm in lead II (Figure 8.2a). Adenosine MPS is performed with normal perfusion at stress and rest (Figure 8.2b). The stress images are displayed on the top row

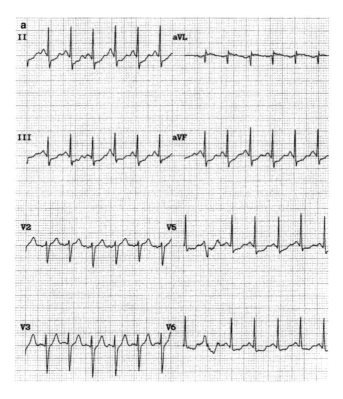

Figure 8.2   *(Continued)*

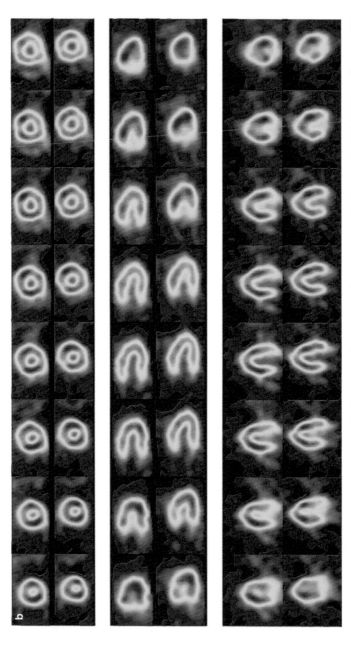

Figure 8.2 Clinical case B. (a) Exercise ECG showing inferolateral ST depression with a maximum of 1.5 mm in lead II. (b) Normal myocardial perfusion at stress and rest. The stress images are displayed on the top row.

Patients with diabetes

The prevalence of type 2 diabetes continues to increase, and it is well known that diabetes confers an increased risk of cardiovascular events. Diabetes increases an individual's risk of heart disease by 2–4 times. In the developed world, half the deaths in the diabetic population are due to heart disease, so this clearly is a big problem.

It is not uncommon for patients with diabetes to be unable to perform a satisfactory exercise test. This is often due to obesity or a general lack of physical fitness. The presence of comorbidities such as peripheral vascular disease or peripheral neuropathy also prevents exercise testing. Furthermore, those with diabetes are more likely to have silent ischaemia, which is detected less accurately by exercise testing than other methods.[16,17] Many diabetic patients with coronary artery disease never have symptoms before presenting with a myocardial infarct, and a quarter of patients presenting with an acute MI prove to have undiagnosed diabetes.

As exercise testing is known to be of lower sensitivity and specificity in individuals with diabetes, pharmacological stress is a more appropriate technique.[17] Reflecting this, NICE have recommended MPS as a first line investigation for suspected CAD in diabetes (Table 8.1). The sensitivity and specificity of MPS in detecting coronary artery disease in the diabetic population is similar to that for non-diabetics. The prognosis of an abnormal scan is worse for a patient with diabetes than for a non-diabetic with the same degree of abnormality, and those with diabetes tend to present with more severe perfusion defects and have a higher incidence of multivessel disease. Women with diabetes are at greater risk of fatal coronary incidents than men, and for any level of perfusion abnormality, a woman is more likely to die a cardiac death than a man. Thus, MPS has an important role to play in the management of heart disease in patients who also have diabetes.[18]

Clinical case C

A 60-year-old female outpatient with diabetes is referred for perfusion imaging due to a history of exertional breathlessness and slight chest discomfort. Examination and resting ECG are normal and she undergoes adenosine stress perfusion imaging. With the infusion of adenosine she experiences chest pain and breathlessness and a fall in systolic blood pressure. Her ECG becomes abnormal (Figure 8.3a) with widespread ST depression. The tracer is injected during pain and her symptoms resolve after the adenosine infusion is stopped. Only stress images are obtained (Figure 8.3b), which show an extensive anteroseptal perfusion defect which extends inferiorly. The polar image (Figure 8.3c), maps the extent of the defect. She is admitted to the coronary care unit directly from the nuclear cardiology department and the decision is made clinically to proceed to urgent coronary angiography without the need for a rest scan. Angiography (Figure 8.3d) demonstrates a severe proximal left anterior descending stenosis which also involves the left main stem (highlighted). She undergoes prompt surgical revascularization during the same admission

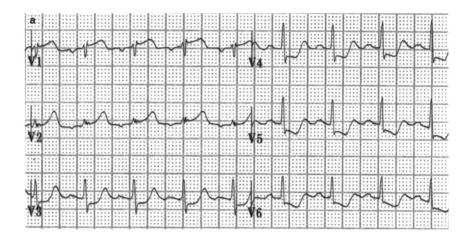

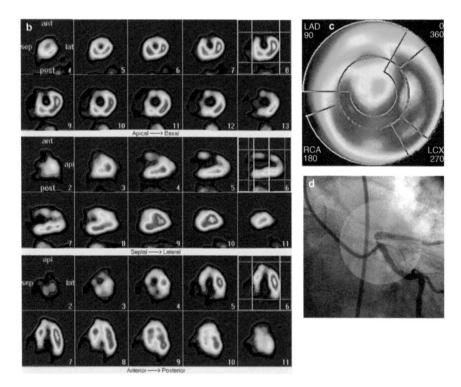

Figure 8.3 Clinical case C. (a) ECG showing widespread ST depression during an adenosine stress test. (b) Perfusion scan images at stress only demonstrating an extensive anteroseptal perfusion defect extending into the inferior territory. (c) Stress polar image mapping the extent of the defect. (d) Coronary angiography demonstrating a severe proximal left anterior descending (LAD) stenosis which also involves the left main stem (highlighted).

REVASCULARIZATION AND MYOCARDIAL PERFUSION SCINTIGRAPHY

MPS is of use both before and after all forms of revascularization (surgery and angioplasty). Many patients are referred for nuclear imaging after angiography to assess the functional significance of observed coronary lesions to determine whether intervention is appropriate. MPS has a role in risk stratification before revascularization. Patients with no inducible defects have a good prognosis with medical treatment even when shown to have three-vessel disease.[19]

MYOCARDIAL PERFUSION SCINTIGRAPHY FOLLOWING PERCUTANEOUS INTERVENTION

MPS is of value in patients with recurrent atypical symptoms following angioplasty. However, in general, MPS should not be performed in the first 6 weeks following PCI. This is because pre-intervention defects may still be present, and in addition the procedure itself causes abnormal endothelial function which may impair coronary flow reserve. Following PCI, a normal scan or the presence of a fixed defect predicts a good prognosis. In contrast, the presence of reversible defects predicts a worse outcome.[20] As well as incomplete revascularization (a residual stenosis) or restenosis, causes of an abnormal scan post-PCI include myocardial infarction during the procedure, side branch occlusion and progression of disease.

Clinical case D

A 52-year-old teacher, with a history of angioplasty and stent insertion for single-vessel LAD disease 3 years earlier, re-presents to the clinic with atypical, though on occasion exertional, chest pain. He was seen 1 year following intervention, with chest discomfort, when he had a negative, high workload, exercise test. His pain remains atypical but is more troublesome. He is anxious that his angina is returning and wonders if he should have an angiogram to check the patency of his stent. On this occasion he undergoes exercise perfusion imaging. He completes four stages of the Bruce protocol without symptoms or ECG changes and his myocardial perfusion scan is normal (Figure 8.4). The images are displayed in standard format with stress images on the upper row. He is reassured and discharged from the clinic

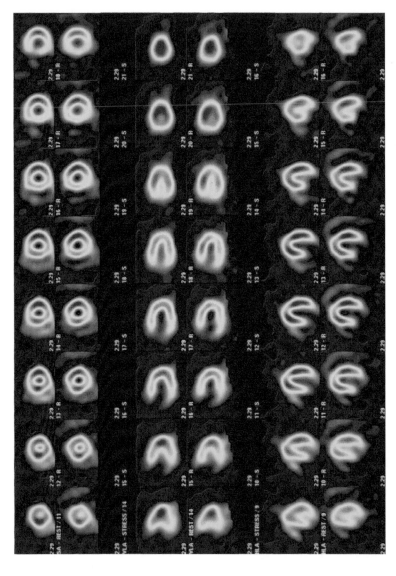

Figure 8.4 Clinical case D. Normal myocardial perfusion scan following 12 minutes' exercise on a treadmill (Bruce protocol).

Clinical case E

A 54-year-old woman presents to the chest pain clinic with typical symptoms of angina. Exercise testing is positive during stage 1 of the Bruce protocol and angiography reveals occlusion of the proximal left anterior descending artery (Figure 8.5a) with backfilling of the LAD (Figure 8.5b arrows) from the right coronary artery. The artery is reopened percutaneously but the final result is suboptimal. Although initially her angina improves, her symptoms recur 2 months later when MPS demonstrates significant anterior reversibility (Figure 8.5c–e: stress images in the upper rows). Repeat angiography shows significant restenosis within the stent (highlighted in Figure 8.5f) and further angioplasty is performed, achieving a good final result (Figure 8.5g)

MYOCARDIAL PERFUSION SCINTIGRAPHY FOLLOWING CORONARY ARTERY BYPASS GRAFTING

MPS is of use following surgical revascularization where there is recurrence of symptoms. Abnormal perfusion may be a result of progression of both native and graft disease, or incomplete revascularization. As is the case after angioplasty, MPS following CABG provides both useful diagnostic and prognostic information, and is better than exercise testing alone.[21]

Clinical case F

CABG is performed on a female patient aged 65 with three-vessel disease (left internal mammary artery (LIMA) to LAD and vein grafts to the right coronary artery and also the posterior descending artery (PDA)). The circumflex is deemed to be too small for successful grafting at the time of operation. Following surgery she continues to have symptoms of angina which are intrusive and myocardial perfusion imaging is performed. The short axis views (Figure 8.6a) and horizontal long axis views (Figure 8.6b) show an inducible defect in the lateral wall. Following successful angioplasty and stenting of the circumflex vessel her symptoms resolve

Clinical case G

A 72-year-old man underwent CABG 7 years ago and re-presents to the clinic with exertional chest pain. His cardiologist carries out an exercise test which is positive, and proceeds to coronary angiography and identifies possible angioplasty targets in the distal native right coronary artery, the native left anterior descending artery, and the graft to the right coronary artery. MPS is requested to assess the functional significance of the stenoses. There is evidence of anterior, lateral and inferior reversibility. Figure 8.7a shows short axis slices and Figure 8.7b vertical long axis slices with the stress images displayed on the upper rows. The patient is offered percutaneous intervention but elects to continue medical therapy

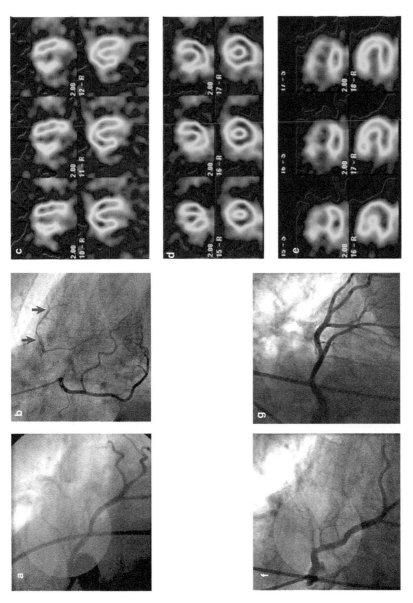

Figure 8.5 Clinical case E. (a) Angiography reveals occlusion of the proximal left anterior descending artery. (b) Angiography showing backfilling of the left anterior descending artery from the right coronary artery (arrows). (c) Horizontal long axis slices demonstrate a reversible defect in the apex and septum. (d) Short axis slices – reversible defect in the anteroseptal territory. (e) Vertical long axis slices at stress demonstrate a significant perfusion defect involving the entire anterior wall and apex with reversibility at rest. The appearances are consistent with a proximal stenosis in the left anterior descending artery (LAD) as demonstrated at angiography. (f) Repeat angiography demonstrating a significant restenosis within the stented LAD (highlighted). (g) A good final result following further intervention to the LAD stenosis.

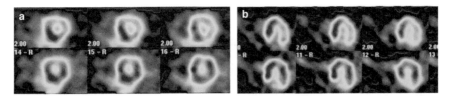

Figure 8.6 Clinical case F. (a) Short axis views demonstrate a reversible defect in the lateral wall. (b) A reversible defect in the lateral wall is clearly demonstrated on the horizontal long axis slices and is consistent with a stenosis in the circumflex vessel.

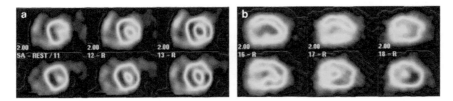

Figure 8.7 Clinical case G. (a, b) Perfusion scan in a 72-year-old male post-coronary artery bypass grafting (CABG) shows evidence of reversibility in the anterior, lateral and inferior territories demonstrated here on the short axis and vertical long axis slices.

ASSESSMENT OF LEFT VENTRICULAR SYSTOLIC FUNCTION

Cardiologists have a choice of non-invasive imaging modalities for assessing left ventricular (LV) function. Unlike echocardiography, radionuclide imaging has the advantage of not relying on assumptions concerning the geometry of the ventricle to calculate chamber volume and ejection fraction (EF). Both radionuclide angiography using multiple gated acquisition (MUGA) or rest-only gated SPECT are techniques which provide highly reproducible measurements of LV function. A further advantage is the fact that measurements can be obtained in virtually all patients, which again is not the case with echocardiography. However, cumulative radiation exposure should be considered where repeated measurements are required, and this is particularly true in children with cancer, where echocardiography is preferred.

In Leeds, we have seen a significant increase in the number of patients requiring regular (3-monthly) monitoring of LV function due to the increased use of trastuzumab (Herceptin®) for both early and advanced breast carcinoma. By working closely with the oncology team we are able to offer a one-stop service, the scan being performed and reported so that the patient can take their current EF result with them to their clinic appointment where they receive the next dose of their chemotherapy. With a little planning it is possible to schedule repeat appointments at 3-monthly intervals. Clearly this practice is not unique to nuclear cardiology – similar arrangements occur in cardiac ultrasound departments, and, as always, local service provision and waiting times will influence which test is used.

We also work with the heart failure service, assessing ventricular function before and after volume reduction surgery and measuring the ejection fraction in patients being investigated for possible AICD (automatic implanted cardiac defibrillator) implantation. The use of gated SPECT in these patients gives information about rest perfusion and wall motion as well as volumes and function.

MYOCARDIAL PERFUSION SCINTIGRAPHY BEFORE NON-CARDIAC SURGERY

We are often asked by surgical or anaesthetic colleagues to comment on a patient's suitability for non-cardiac surgery, usually in patients with known or suspected heart disease. We have found that developing close links between the department and the referrers – especially the vascular surgery and renal transplant teams – allows discussion about which investigation is required. Once again this is where the involvement of a cardiologist in your nuclear cardiology department is a definite bonus. Unnecessary tests can be avoided, and the patient receives appropriate investigation and risk reduction measures. In some cases, review of the patient and their notes can provide the necessary risk assessment and avoid the need for a visit to the department for the patient. For example, those patients who only have minor clinical predictors of risk (including advanced age, previous stroke, abnormal resting ECG or hypertension) who require low- or moderate-risk surgery do not require further investigation.[22]

With appropriate patient selection, MPS provides useful prognostic information in patients who are to undergo non-cardiac surgery. Asymptomatic patients who have a low risk of coronary disease do not require perfusion imaging to look for silent ischaemia. In this patient group the event rate is very low, and most events will occur after a normal scan.[23]

MPS is appropriate for those patients who are at intermediate clinical risk (for example, diabetics, those with stable angina or controlled heart failure) and who are due to undergo intermediate- or high-risk surgery. The predictive value of a normal scan is particularly high (96%). Where there is evidence suggesting ischaemia the positive predictive value is low, but unsurprisingly those patients with reversible defects pose a greater risk that those with fixed defects. As one would expect, those with LV impairment are also at increased risk. There is, however, no evidence to support the use of prophylactic revascularization, and the decision to perform CABG or PCI is made using the same criteria as in patients who are not candidates for non-cardiac surgery – there must be a good clinical indication for intervention. Modern anaesthetics and the use of beta blockade, aggressive risk factor modification, and invasive monitoring all serve to reduce the risk of perioperative events, and our

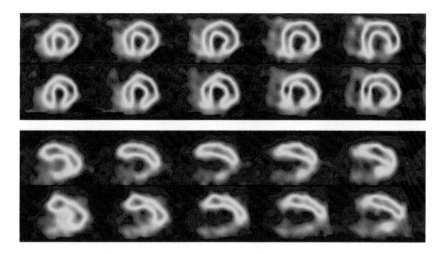

Figure 8.8   Clinical case H. Myocardial perfusion scintigraphy reveals a fixed defect in the inferior wall consistent with a previous occlusion to the right coronary artery. The findings are supported by the gated single photon emission computed tomography (SPECT) images where the inferior wall is found to be hypokinetic on wall motion analysis.

vascular anaesthetists know the importance of booking an intensive care bed for the higher-risk patients.

Clinical case H

A 65-year-old man with a history of a previous angioplasty and stent insertion to the right coronary artery who also has end-stage renal failure and type 2 diabetes is referred for perfusion imaging as part of his work-up for renal transplantation. He is free of cardiovascular symptoms and is on appropriate secondary preventive medication. His ECG shows inferior Q waves and adenosine perfusion imaging is performed; his scan (Figure 8.8) shows a fixed inferior defect demonstrated here on the vertical long axis view, but is otherwise normal. Gated imaging reveals a normal sized ventricle, an ejection fraction of 50% and inferior hypokinesis in keeping with a previous inferior infarct. On this basis he is accepted on the transplant list

---

MYOCARDIAL PERFUSION SCINTIGRAPHY AND VOCATIONAL DRIVING LICENSING

The UK Driver and Vehicle Licensing Authority (DVLA) requires cardiovascular assessment before issuing Group 2 licences for drivers of buses and lorries and other professional drivers (previously characterized as heavy goods vehicle and public service vehicle (HGV and PSV) drivers). Patients with a history of coronary artery disease, significant peripheral vascular disease (including surgery for aortic aneurysms) and previous cerebrovascular disease are required to undergo cardiac assessment.[24]

The standard DVLA requirement is satisfactory completion of three stages of a Bruce protocol treadmill test without symptoms or signs of cardiac dysfunction and no significant ST segment change on the ECG, and no malignant dysrhythmia or claudication. The test should be performed off all antianginal therapy for 48 hours. Many individuals are unable to complete 9 minutes on the treadmill, and some will have resting ECG abnormalities making exercise testing difficult to interpret (bundle branch block and other conduction defects). In addition, some patients following revascularization can complete the exercise requirements, but have persistently abnormal ECG tracings despite the absence of symptoms and good angiographic results. Increasingly the DVLA are using MPS as a means to assess fitness to hold a vocational licence. As with standard treadmill testing, the DVLA have a recommended protocol, and gated SPECT is required. To fulfil licensing criteria, any inducible perfusion defect must involve less than 10% of the myocardium. In addition, the LVEF must be greater than 40%.[24]

With the more widespread use of MPS by the DVLA, patients are not being disadvantaged by the reliance on treadmill testing, which is inappropriate for many of them. Many drivers are now re-licenced on the basis of a satisfactory perfusion scan, where previously they would have lost their vocational licence on the basis of an inadequate exercise test. In Leeds we have seen a steady increase in the number of patients referred to us by the DVLA, many of them coming from outside our immediate region.

Clinical case I

A 50-year-old HGV driver undergoes three-vessel CABG for angina. Treadmill testing for relicensing is performed. He is completely asymptomatic and completes three stages of the Bruce protocol without chest pain, but the ECG shows 2 mm lateral ST depression (Figure 8.9) seen in leads V5 and V6. Pre-revascularization, his exercise treadmill test (ETT) had been positive early in stage 2 for both symptoms and significant ST depression. On this basis, Group 2 licensing is refused by the DVLA. His cardiologist considers that his ETT is abnormal due to surgery (as is often the case), and coronary and graft angiography reveal patent grafts. Gated MPS is performed which shows normal perfusion at both stress and rest, and the ejection fraction is 54%. On the basis of this study the DVLA permit relicensing

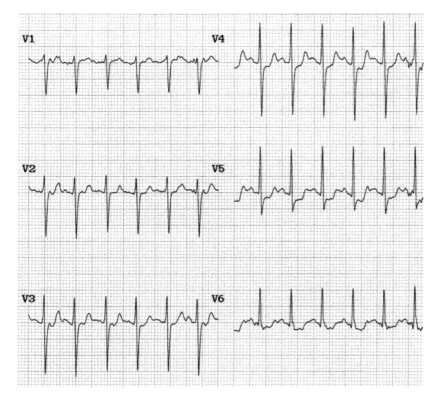

Figure 8.9 Clinical case I. Treadmill testing in a 50-year-old heavy goods vehicle (HGV) driver reveals 2-mm lateral ST depression in leads V5 and V6.

CONCLUSION

This has been a relatively brief review of the role of MPS in clinical management from the cardiologist's point of view. Here, and in preceding chapters, we have emphasised the need for close cooperation between the nuclear cardiology department and the referring cardiologists, and there is no doubt that where this can be achieved it has a beneficial effect on quality, and facilitates the smooth running of the department. The principles outlined have allowed us to provide a service which cardiologists have found useful, and we have seen referrals increasing steadily, although achievement of the NICE target is still some way off. However, there is always more you can do, and in addition to maintaining the upward trend in referrals, we are keen to introduce a walk-in (or wheel-in) service for the acute chest pain clinic. Who knows, we may need to think about an on-call and weekend service as part of the

24/7 hospital. In the mean time, we hope this book will have been useful for readers who are just starting out in nuclear cardiology.

APPENDIX

Useful website addresses

www.acc.org	American Heart Association
www.asnc.org	American Society of Nuclear Cardiology
www.bncs.org.uk	British Nuclear Cardiology Society
www.bnms.org.uk	British Nuclear Medicine Society
www.eanm.org	European Association of Nuclear Medicine
www.escardio.org	European Society of Cardiology
www.snm.org	Society of Nuclear Medicine
www.dvla.gov.uk/medical.aspx	Driver and Vehicle Licensing Authority
www.nice.org.uk	National Institute for Health and Clinical Excellence

REFERENCES

1. Underwood SR, Anagnostopoulos C, Cerquiera M et al. Myocardial perfusion scintigraphy: the evidence. Eur J Nucl Med 2004; 31: 261–91.
2. Flocke FJ et al. ACC/AHA/ASNC Guidelines for the clinical use of cardiac radionuclide imaging. American College of Cardiology, 2003. (online at http//www.acc.org/clinical-guidelines/radio/rni_fulltext.pdf).
3. Anagnostopoulos C, Harbinson M, Kelion A et al. Procedure guidelines for radionuclide myocardial perfusion imaging. Heart 2004; 90 (Suppl I): i1–10.
4. Underwood SR, Godman B, Salyani JR et al. Economics of Myocardial Perfusion Imaging in Europe – the EMPIRE study. Eur Heart J 1999; 20: 157–66.
5. National Institute for Health and Clinical Excellence. Myocardial perfusion scintigraphy for the diagnosis and management of angina and myocardial infarction. Technology Appraisal Guidance 73, November 2003.
6. Iskander S, Iskandrian AE. Risk assessment using single-photon emission computed tomographic technetium-99m sestamibi imaging. J Am Coll Cardiol 1998; 32: 57–62.
7. de Bono D. Investigation and management of stable angina: revised guidelines 1998. Heart 1999; 81: 546–55.
8. Fox K, Garcia MA, Ardissino D et al. Guidelines on the management of stable angina pectoris: executive summary: the Task Force on the Management of Stable Angina Pectoris of the European Society of Cardiology. Eur Heart J 2006; 27: 1341–81.
9. Kelion A, Anagnostopoulos C, Harbinson M et al. Myocardial perfusion scintigraphy in the UK: insights from the British Nuclear Cardiology Society survey 2000. Heart 2005; 91 (Suppl IV): iv2–6.

10. Bateman TM, Pruvlovich E. Assessment of prognosis in chronic coronary heart disease. Heart 2004; 90 (Suppl V): v10–15.

11. Bax JJ, van der Wall EE, Harbinson MT. Radionuclide techniques for the assessment of myocardial viability and hibernation. Heart 2004; 90 (Suppl V): v26–33.

12. Underwood SR, Shaw LJ. Myocardial perfusion scintigraphy and cost effectiveness of diagnosis and management of coronary heart disease. Heart 2004; 90 (Suppl V): v34–6.

13. Mieres JH. Review of the American Heart Association's guidelines for cardiovascular disease prevention in women. Heart 2006; 92 (Suppl III): iii10–13.

14. Detry JM, Kapita BM, Cosyms J et al. Diagnostic value of history and maximal exercise electrocardiography in men and women suspected of coronary heart disease. Circulation 1977; 55: 756–61.

15. Kennedy JW, Killip T, Fisher LD et al. The clinical spectrum of coronary artery disease and its surgical and medical management, 1974–1979. The Coronary Artery Surgery Study. Circulation 1982; 66: 16–23.

16. Iskandrian AE, Heo J, Nallamothu N. Detection of coronary artery disease in women with use of stress single-photon emission computed tomography myocardial perfusion imaging. J Nucl Cardiol 1997; 4: 329–35.

17. Zellweger MJ, Hachamovitch R, Kang X et al. Prognostic relevance of symptoms versus objective evidence of coronary artery disease in diabetic patients. Eur Heart J 2004; 25: 543–50.

18. Giri S, Shaw LJ, Murthy DR et al. Impact of diabetes on the risk stratification using stress single-photon emission computed tomography myocardial perfusion imaging in patients with symptoms suggestive of coronary artery disease. Circulation 2002; 105: 32–40.

19. Brown KA, Rowen M. Prognostic value of a normal exercise myocardial perfusion imaging study in patients with angiographically significant coronary artery disease. Am J Cardiol 1993; 71: 865–7.

20. Milan K, Myslivecek M Kvarilova M et al. Prognostic value of myocardial perfusion tomographic imaging in patients after percutaneous transluminal coronary angioplasty. Clin Nucl Med 2000; 25: 775–8.

21. Lauer MS, Lytle B, Pashkow F et al. Prediction of death and myocardial infarction by screening with exercise thallium testing after coronary artery bypass grafting. Lancet 1998; 351: 615–22.

22. Eagle KA, Berger PB, Calkins H et al. ACC/AHA guideline update on perioperative cardiovascular evaluation for non cardiac surgery. Circulation 2002; 105: 1257–67.

23. Fleg JL, Gerstneblisth G, Zonderman AB et al. Prevalence and prognostic significance of exercise induced silent myocardial ischaemia detected by thallium scintigraphy and electrocardiography in asymptomatic volunteers. Circulation 1990; 81; 428–36.

24. Drivers Medical Group. At a glance guide to the current standards of fitness to drive. Swansea: DVLA, 2007.

Index

Page numbers in *italics* refer to tables and figures.

Printed and bound by CPI Group (UK) Ltd, Croydon, CR0 4YY

23/10/2024

01778263-0018